Fast-track Strategies for Navigating Abuse

Setting Boundaries and Healing Relationships

Susan Beaumont

Copyright © 2024 Susan Beaumont. All rights reserved.

The content within this book may not be reproduced, duplicated, or transmitted without direct written permission from the author or the publisher.

Under no circumstances will any blame or legal responsibility be held against the publisher, or author, for any damages, reparation, or monetary loss due to the information contained within this book, either directly or indirectly.

Legal Notice:

This book is copyright protected. It is only for personal use. You cannot amend, distribute, sell, use, quote, or paraphrase any part of the content within this book, without the consent of the author or publisher.

Disclaimer Notice:

Please note the information contained within this document is for educational and entertainment purposes only. All effort has been expended to present accurate, up-to-date, reliable, and complete information. No warranties of any kind are declared or implied. Readers acknowledge that the author is not engaged in the rendering of legal, financial, medical, or professional advice. The content within this book has been derived from various sources. Please consult a licensed professional before attempting any techniques outlined in this book.

By reading this document, the reader agrees that under no circumstances is the author responsible for any losses, direct or indirect, that are incurred as a result of the use of the information contained within this document, including, but not limited to, errors, omissions, or inaccuracies.

Contents

Introduction	5
1. Decoding Narcissism	7
2. Recognizing Abuse and Its Impact	25
3. Strategies for Emotional Protection	41
4. Setting and Enforcing Boundaries	59
5. Advanced Strategies for High-Conflict Situations	69
6. Recovery	73
7. Practical Advice for Exiting Toxic Relationships	89
8. Healing and Moving Forward	103
Conclusion	135
References	139

Introduction

Once radiating joy, I was now frequently anxious and unsure. This wasn't just a rough patch; it was the devastating impact of living with a partner whose narcissistic tendencies slowly eroded my sense of self. This moment isn't just my story—it's shared by many, perhaps by you too. It's a painful reminder of the destructive power of narcissistic journey to reclaiming one's life.

Narcissism, in its essence, is characterized by an inflated sense of self-importance, a deep need for excessive attention and admiration, and a lack of empathy for others. However, the effects on relationships are far more profound than the simple definitions suggest. Whether overt or covert, the narcissist in your life can leave you feeling isolated, worthless, and utterly confused. It is a form of emotional and psychological manipulation that can leave deep scars.

This book is born from a deep-seated desire to light a path to recovery for those who feel lost in the shadows of narcissistic abuse. With over four decades of experience in administration, focusing mainly on supporting vulnerable populations, I've witnessed the resilience of the human spirit. My work, from developing statewide projects to fight poverty to leading initiatives to end homelessness, has shown me the power of community and support in overcoming adversity. Now, I turn this focus to you—the survivors and warriors of hidden battles in personal relationships.

"Unmask Narcissism: Fast-Track Relationship Recovery Strategies" is not just a book; it's a lifeline. Here, you will find a blend of professional advice and compassionate empathy, all aimed at guiding you through recognizing narcissistic behaviors, surviving and leaving toxic relationships, and, most importantly, healing. We'll explore the importance of establishing self-love boundaries, cultivating resilience, and reclaiming emotional health.

As you turn these pages, you should view this as more than just reading. Engage with the content, reflect on your experiences, and apply the strategies discussed. Each chapter is designed to address different facets of narcissistic abuse and recovery, providing you with a comprehensive roadmap from recognizing the signs to nurturing your recovery.

You will not be alone in this journey. Through heartfelt stories, practical advice, and supportive insights, this book will stand as a beacon of hope and empowerment. Together, we will navigate the complex terrain of emotional healing and celebrate each step toward freedom and personal growth.

As we embark on this journey together, remember that healing is possible and within your reach. Let this book be your guide back to yourself, to a life filled with joy, respect, and love—a life you truly deserve.

Chapter 1
Decoding Narcissism

Have you ever had that moment when you're watching a movie, and the charming, seemingly perfect character slowly begins to reveal a less savory side? It's a plot twist we didn't see coming but one that feels all too real for those who have experienced life with a narcissist. Understanding narcissism, particularly its spectrum from overt to covert, is like peeling back the layers of an onion. Each layer offers more insight, sometimes making you want to cry. In this chapter, we'll explore these layers, offering you, not just insight but tools to recognize and cope with narcissistic behaviors in your own life.

1.1 The Spectrum of Narcissism: From Overt to Covert

Let's start by setting the stage with what narcissism entails. Picture a spectrum. On one end, there's overt narcissism, which is the kind you probably picture when you hear the term "narcissist." It's the grandiose, attention-seeking, and overtly self-confident behavior that can be as blatant as a neon sign. On the opposite end lies covert narcissism, which is trickier to detect. These individuals still crave admiration and importance but in a much quieter, perhaps even shy, manner.

Definition and Differentiation

From what I have gathered, narcissism is rooted in Narcissistic Personality Disorder (NPD), a mental condition characterized by a long-term pattern of exaggerated feelings of self-importance, an excessive need for admiration, and a lack of empathy toward other people. Where overt narcissists might openly demand admiration and attention, covert narcissists do so in more subtle, indirect ways. They may play the victim or use passive-aggressiveness as a tool, making them harder to identify than their overt counterparts.

Behavioral Characteristics

Overt narcissists are often the life of the party. They seek the spotlight and feel entitled to it. Their arrogance can be off-putting to some, but it comes off as charismatic confidence to others. They might interrupt conversations to turn the focus onto themselves and will often exaggerate their achievements. Covert narcissists, by contrast, might not openly seek the spotlight, but they are equally hungry for admiration. They might sulk or withdraw if they feel they're not getting the attention they deserve or manipulate situations subtly to gain sympathy and praise.

For example, consider an overt narcissist at a work meeting. They might boldly claim credit for a team's success, overshadowing the contributions of others. A covert narcissist in the same setting might quietly imply their pivotal role in the project's success, hinting at obstacles they overcame and making others feel compelled to offer the recognition they crave.

Impact on Relationships

The emotional toll on relationships may be profound, regardless of whether narcissism is overt or covert. Overt narcissists may openly belittle their partners to maintain a sense of superiority. Family dinners could become platforms for their achievements, where others feel diminished or ignored. Covert narcissists, on the other hand, might manipulate loved ones through guilt. Imagine a partner who perpetually plays the victim, suggesting that you don't spend enough time with them, subtly suggesting their needs aren't met because of your actions.

Identification Tips

Identifying whether someone is displaying narcissistic tendencies involves observing how they react to various situations. Red flags for overt narcissism include a palpable need for admiration, a propensity to talk about themselves incessantly, and visible discomfort or irritation when they are not the center of attention. For covert narcissism, look for subtle signs of passive-aggressive behavior, a tendency to play the victim, or a pattern of manipulating others' emotions to gain sympathy or support.

Recognizing these signs early is crucial for managing personal boundaries and protecting your emotional well-being. As we peel back the layers of narcissism's impact, understanding these behaviors empowers you to navigate these complex dynamics more effectively, whether in personal relationships, professional settings, or social interactions.

1.2 Psychological Profiles: Understanding the Narcissist's Mind

Have you ever wondered what goes on in a narcissist's mind? It's like trying to understand a foreign language without a translator. In this section, we explore the psychological makeup of narcissists, their cognitive functioning, and their emotional landscape and uncover why their manipulation tactics are so darn effective. Understanding these aspects can be like finally getting that translator who helps you understand the language.

Cognitive Functioning

Narcissists often view the world in black and white. This polarized way of thinking simplifies complex human behavior into good or bad, right or wrong, with or against them. It's a cognitive bias that feeds their need for superiority. If they're always 'right,' anyone who disagrees or challenges them must be 'wrong.' This isn't just frustrating; it's a fundamental component of their psyche. Psychological theories suggest that this divided thinking pattern stems from early childhood experiences where ambiguity and uncertainty were met with disdain or punishment, leading to a rigid cognitive style that craves order and disdains complexity.

Another cornerstone of the narcissistic cognitive style is the superiority complex. It's not just about feeling superior; it's about needing to feel superior to avoid the crushing weight of their insecurities. Studies, such as those in the realm of social psychology, have shown that narcissists' grandiose self-view is a shield against deep-seated feelings of inadequacy. This mental conflict—they are the best, yet they fear they are the worst—is a tightrope they walk every day.

Emotional Landscape

A narcissist's emotions are often contradictory. They have a vast need for admiration and a barren lack of empathy for others. This emotional setup is like a garden that only grows thistles. The lack of empathy isn't just a lack of concern for others' feelings; it's an inability to recognize those feelings as legitimate or genuine. It's why a narcissist can hurt you deeply and not understand why you're upset. They're not wired to connect their actions with your emotional responses.

Underneath their exterior, narcissists harbor profound insecurities. These are not the common insecurities everyone experiences. For narcissists, these insecurities deeply affect their sense of self, which relies heavily on external validation. Without this validation, their self-esteem doesn't just wobble—it crumbles. Psychological research on narcissism often highlights this fragile self-esteem as a core feature of both overt and covert forms of the disorder.

Manipulation Tactics

Understanding the narcissist's manipulation tactics is akin to a magician revealing his secrets. Once you see the mechanics, the illusion loses its power. Narcissists are adept at reading others to discern their desires and fears. This keen observation allows them to tailor their manipulations precisely to the individual, making their tactics particularly effective. They might use flattery, promises, or stoking fears to maneuver others into positions that bolster their sense of superiority and control.

The psychological basis for why these tactics work is rooted in basic human needs for acceptance and fear of abandonment.

Narcissists exploit these needs by positioning themselves as the granter of love and approval while simultaneously threatening withdrawal. It's a powerful combination that can bind people to them, clouding judgment and overriding rational thought.

Defense Mechanisms

Narcissists are champions at employing defense mechanisms to protect their fragile egos. Denial and projection are among their favorites. Denial allows them to refuse acknowledgment of any personal flaw. If you raise a concern about their behavior, they'll likely rebut with complete denial that the behavior is anything but perfect. Projection, on the other hand, involves attributing undesirable traits to others. If they're feeling insecure, they might accuse you of being insecure instead.

These mechanisms do more than just protect their ego; they warp reality. For those in a relationship with a narcissist, this can lead to a disorienting world where nothing is quite as it seems. Understanding these defenses can equip you with the knowledge to see through the distortions and recognize the tactics for what they are—a desperate attempt to maintain a veneer of perfection.

Exploring the inner workings of a narcissist's mind is more than just an academic exercise. It's a crucial step in understanding the dynamics of your interactions with them. With this understanding, you can better protect your emotional health and make informed relationship decisions.

1.3 Gaslighting and Its Discontents: A Close Look at Manipulative Tactics

Gaslighting, a term that has seeped into our everyday vocabulary, often pops up in discussions about psychological manipulation. But what does it mean? The concept originated from the 1938 play "Gas Light," where a husband manipulates his wife into believing she's losing her sanity. Today, it refers to a form of psychological abuse where a person or a group covertly sows seeds of doubt in a targeted individual, making them question their memory, perception, or judgment. It's a clever move favored by narcissists because it taps directly into the psyche of their victims, rendering them more pliable and less likely to challenge the narcissist's authority or version of events.

Imagine you're in a relationship where you recount an incident or conversation, and the response is always a denial or a twisted version that makes you question your sanity. "That's not how it happened; you're always making things up!" is a classic gaslighting response. Here, the manipulator not only dismisses the claim but also counterattacks, making the victim question their reality and often their mental stability. This tactic is exceptionally gradual because it creates doubt and isolates the victim, usually making them reliant on the gaslighter for their version of 'reality.'

The psychological effects of being gaslighted are profound. In the short term, victims may experience confusion, anxiety, and a crippling sense of self-doubt. They might find themselves constantly apologizing, over-explaining simple decisions, or unable to make decisions without excessive reassurance from others. Long-term effects can be even more damaging, including a significant loss of self-esteem, persistent anxiety, and even depression. Victims may also develop a form of learned helplessness. In this state, they are conditioned to believe they have no control over their situation, which can permeate all aspects of their lives, making recovery and escape from the abusive environment all the more challenging.

To counteract gaslighting, the first step is to recognize it. This can be challenging, especially when you're in the thick of it, but there are signs. Keep an eye out for patterns of behavior where your feelings are consistently minimized or dismissed or where your emotional reactions are used against you ("You're too sensitive!" or "You have no sense of humor!"). Documentation can help solidify your reality—keep a journal of incidents that felt 'off' to you, noting what was said and how it made you think. This record can be a grounding tool when you start to doubt your memory or perception.

Another effective strategy is establishing a network of trust outside the narcissist's influence. This could be friends, family, or a therapist who knows your history and can validate your experiences and feelings. This network helps affirm your reality and provides emotional support, which is crucial for anyone attempting to break free from the cycle of manipulation. Finally, when possible, setting clear boundaries with the gaslighter is vital. This means limiting what topics you discuss with them or engaging only in the presence of others, which can mitigate some of the gaslighter's power over your reality.

Understanding the mechanics behind gaslighting and learning strategies to counter its effects can empower you to reclaim your sense of self and move towards a healthier, more autonomous life. Remember, the goal isn't just to survive these encounters; it's to thrive beyond them with a renewed trust in yourself and your perception of the world around you.

1.4 The Narcissistic Cycle: Idealization, Devaluation, and Discard

Understanding the narcissistic cycle is like getting a behind-the-scenes tour of a magic show. The illusion loses its power once you know how the tricks are done. This cycle, consisting of idealization, devaluation, and discard, is a manipulative whirlwind designed to hook and destabilize the victim, ensuring they are malleable and overly dependent on the narcissist's approval and affection. Recognizing and breaking free from this cycle can be as liberating as it is challenging.

Cycle Explanation

The cycle starts with **idealization.** In this phase, the narcissist showers their target with excessive admiration and compliments, fast-tracking intimacy and connection. It's like being hit by a love bomb. You may feel you've met your soulmate, as they align perfectly with your deepest desires and needs. Psychologically, this phase exploits your natural response to reciprocal affection and bonding. The narcissist studies and mirrors your likes, dislikes, and even your deepest insecurities to position themselves as the perfect partner or friend.

Next comes **devaluation.** Once the narcissist feels secure in their hold over you, their attitude shifts dramatically. The compliments turn to criticism, the intimacy into indifference. Suddenly, you find yourself on an emotional seesaw, desperately trying to regain the affection and approval you once received in abundance. This phase is marked by frequent belittling, gaslighting, and manipulation, aiming to erode your self-esteem and increase your reliance on the narcissist. The psychological tactic here is to keep you unsteady and off-kilter, thereby asserting their dominance and control.

The final phase is **discard.** This phase occurs when the narcissist decides you are no longer applicable to their needs, and they may abandon the relationship in a cold, calculated way. Depending on their needs or current options, it can be temporary or permanent. The discard is especially traumatic as it comes after intense emotional or psychological investment, leaving you feeling used, worthless, and confused.

Phase-Specific Behaviors

During **idealization**, the narcissist might present behaviors like constant texting or calling, extravagant gestures, and declarations of love or deep connection early on. They appear attentive and interested in everything about you, making you feel like the center of their world. In contrast, **devaluation** manifests through actions such as withdrawing affection, ignoring your emotional needs, criticizing harshly, or being passive-aggressive. They might compare you unfavorably to others or blame you for their problematic behaviors, shifting the goalposts constantly to ensure you can never feel secure or competent.

When the **discard** phase hits, the narcissist may cut off contact suddenly, become involved with someone else without previous indication, or simply show indifference towards your feelings. They might block you on social media, refuse to answer calls, or even spread malicious gossip to mutual acquaintances.

Impact on the Victim

Navigating through these phases can feel like riding the worst emotional rollercoaster. The **idealization** phase can make you feel incredibly valued and loved, setting a psychological standard you strive to maintain or reclaim long after it's gone. When **devaluation** starts, it can induce significant emotional confusion and distress. You may question your worth, over-analyze your behavior, and feel desperate to fix things, not realizing that the deck is systematically stacked against you.

The **discard** phase often leaves profound psychological scars, reinforcing feelings of inadequacy and rejection. Victims might struggle with feelings of abandonment, low self-esteem, and even depression. The whiplash from being idolized to devalued and eventually discarded can impact mental health long after the relationship ends.

Breaking the Cycle

Breaking free from this cycle involves recognition, self-reassurance, and establishing firm boundaries. Start by educating yourself about these phases, as you are doing now, which will help you detach from the personal hurt and view these behaviors as symptomatic of the narcissist's personality disorder, not a reflection of your worth.

Documenting interactions can help you maintain a factual basis for what you're experiencing, which is invaluable when your emotions and memories are gaslighted. Lean on supportive friends or family, and consider professional help to navigate out of this cycle. Therapy, particularly with professionals who understand narcissistic abuse, can provide not only a safe space to heal but also tools to rebuild your self-esteem and resilience.

Understanding the narcissistic cycle demystifies the chaos and confusion wrought by such relationships. It arms you with knowledge and strategies to protect yourself and reclaim your autonomy, ensuring you are prepared to close the curtain on this act of the show.

1.5 Subtle Signs: Unmasking Covert Narcissism in Daily Interactions

Navigating the murky waters of covert narcissism can feel like trying to read a book with half the pages missing. The signs are not always clear-cut, and the behaviors can be so subtle that you question your perceptions. Think of covert narcissism as the silent undertow beneath calm waters, powerful enough to pull you under without a single wave in sight. Here, we'll explore some of the subtler signs of covert narcissism, focusing on communication cues, behavior in social versus private settings, reactions to criticism, and emotional manipulation tactics.

Subtleties in Communication

Covert narcissists are masters of indirect communication. Their language is often ambiguous, leaving enough room for plausible deniability while planting seeds of doubt or guilt. Consider passive-aggressiveness one of their go-to tactics. Imagine a scenario where you spend the evening catching up with an old friend instead of your partner. A covert narcissist might respond, "Oh, I'm sure your friend will appreciate your time much more than I would." On the surface, it sounds supportive, but the underlying message is designed to make you feel guilty for choosing someone else over them.

Backhanded compliments are another stealth tool in their arsenal. Picture being congratulated on a professional achievement with a twist that subtly undermines you, such as, "Wow, they're lowering the standards if you got promoted!" It sounds like a compliment, but it's laced with an insult. These communication subtleties serve as critical indicators, hinting at the manipulative undercurrents that define covert narcissism.

Behavior in Social Settings

Covert narcissists often present a charming, even empathetic persona in social settings. This public face can be remarkably different from the one they wear in private. At a party, they might be the attentive listener who laughs at your jokes and seems genuinely interested in your well-being. However, this façade usually crumbles once they're in a more private setting. They might become cold, dismissive, or indifferent to your needs at home.

This stark contrast can be confusing and is often intentionally so. It isolates you from seeking validation of your experiences from others who only see the charming side. It's like living with two different people, making you question your judgment. If you notice such drastic changes in behavior between public and private interactions, take it as a red flag.

Reaction to Criticism

How a person handles criticism can reveal a lot about their character. Covert narcissists typically react poorly to criticism, regardless of how constructive it is. Instead of openly displaying aggression, as an overt narcissist might, the covert narcissist will often employ subtler tactics. For instance, they might sulk, withdraw affection, or engage in silent treatment as punishment. Over time, this can condition you to avoid critiquing them altogether, thereby maintaining their sense of control.

Another common reaction is turning the criticism around to focus on your flaws instead of addressing the feedback. If you are concerned about their behavior, they might respond, "You're just too sensitive." This effectively deflects the criticism and makes it about your supposed overreaction. This allows them to escape accountability and plants seeds of self-doubt within them.

Emotional Manipulation

Emotional manipulation is the covert narcissist's bread and butter. They are adept at manipulating emotions to elicit pity, guilt, or sympathy, which they use to their advantage. One subtle tactic is the victim's stance. They might share stories of their difficult childhood or a previous abusive relationship, tailored in a way that justifies any questionable behavior on their part. The goal is to garner sympathy and frame their negative behaviors as justifiable reactions to past traumas.

Another manipulation technique involves inconsistency in their emotional responses. This unpredictability can keep you off-balance, as you may constantly try to gauge moods or anticipate reactions. Today, they might react to a comment with laughter;

tomorrow, the same comment could provoke sullen silence or a cutting remark. This tactic is not just confusing—it's designed to keep you in a state of perpetual anxiety about how they will react, making it easier for them to control you.

Understanding these subtle signs is crucial in recognizing and handling interactions with a covert narcissist. It's about reading between the lines and seeing beyond the façade. This knowledge arms you with the ability to maintain your boundaries and protect your emotional health against the often invisible yet profoundly impactful manipulations of a covert narcissist.

1.6 Narcissistic Triggers: What Sets Them Off and Why?

Understanding what triggers a narcissist can feel akin to walking through a minefield with a blindfold. You never quite know when you might step on a trigger that sets off an explosive reaction. It's daunting but not incomprehensible. Narcissists, with their fragile egos and constant need for admiration, react to perceived threats or slights with behaviors that can range from cold withdrawal to aggressive confrontation. Knowing these triggers, why they are so potent, and how to manage them can transform your interactions from a nerve-wracking game of chance into a more predictable, manageable experience.

Common Triggers

Narcissists are often triggered by anything that they perceive as a threat to their ego or self-esteem. This could be as overt as public criticism or as subtle as not receiving the expected attention or praise. For example, if you were to commend a colleague openly for their contribution to a project in which a narcissist was also involved, it might trigger a reaction. The narcissist might see this as sidelining or undervaluing their contribution, even if the intention was purely to give credit where it was due.

Other common triggers include perceived betrayal or disloyalty and situations where they feel they have lost control. A narcissist wants to be seen as the leader, the best, the infallible. Any hint of dissent, such as someone disagreeing with them in a meeting or not following their advice, can be seen as challenging their authority and thus trigger an adverse reaction.

Psychological Background

The potency of these triggers lies in the narcissist's fragile self-worth. Psychologically, narcissists have a distorted self-image. Their external facade of superiority and confidence masks a deep-seated sense of insecurity and inadequacy. Psychological theories suggest that this is often rooted in early developmental experiences where their inherent worth was conditional upon achievements or specific behaviors, leading them to seek validation to feel worthy constantly.

When something happens that contradicts their self-image—like someone else receiving praise or not getting their way—it creates an emotional struggle. They face a direct conflict between the reality they encounter and the inflated self-image they strive to maintain. Their typical reaction is not to adjust their self-perception but to alter or attack the source of the contradiction. This is why their responses to such triggers can be extreme and disproportionate.

Examples of Triggered Behaviors

When triggered, narcissists' behaviors can vary widely, but they typically involve some form of aggression or withdrawal designed to reaffirm their sense of superiority. For instance, if a narcissist feels upstaged at work, they might react by belittling their colleague's ideas in future meetings to undermine them and reestablish their dominance. Alternatively, they might withdraw and give their colleague the silent treatment, refusing to communicate effectively as a form of punishment and control.

In personal relationships, a narcissist might react to perceived criticism by lashing out, accusing the other person of being ungrateful or incompetent, or they might play the victim, twisting the situation to make it appear that they are the one who has been wronged. This deflects the focus from their flaws and manipulates the other person into reassurance and apology, thus feeding the narcissist's need for emotional nourishment.

Handling Triggers

Dealing with a triggered narcissist requires a delicate balance of assertiveness and tact. First and foremost, it's crucial to maintain calm. Reacting emotionally only escalates conflicts and plays into the narcissist's hands, giving them the drama and attention they crave. Instead, respond with measured, controlled statements acknowledging their feelings but not conceding your boundaries. For instance, if a narcissist reacts negatively to praise you've given someone else, you might say, "I understand you feel overlooked, and I value your contributions as well. Let's find a time to discuss your role in more detail."

Setting clear boundaries is also essential. This doesn't mean cutting off all interaction but defining what behavior you will not tolerate and sticking to it. Suppose a narcissist starts to belittle you during a triggered episode; calmly but firmly state that you are willing to discuss the matter respectfully and are not willing to continue the conversation otherwise. Establishing a mutual understanding of boundaries between the narcissist and the victim is crucial for managing the narcissist's behavior.

Lastly, provide reassurance of their value without unduly feeding their ego. This can be a nuanced approach, where you acknowledge their feelings or contributions without excessive praise. It's about striking a balance that keeps the peace without reinforcing unhealthy dynamics.

Navigating life with a narcissist, be it at work or in personal relationships, is undeniably challenging. By understanding what triggers narcissistic behaviors and learning how to respond effectively, you can create a less volatile, more harmonious interaction. It's about protecting your emotional well-being while tactfully managing theirs, ensuring your interactions are as constructive and peaceful as possible. Remember, while you may not be able to change a narcissist, you can change how you interact with them, and sometimes, that can make all the difference.

Chapter 2
Recognizing Abuse and Its Impact

Have you ever felt like you're living in a fog, unsure if your feelings are valid or if your experiences are just a series of overreactions? It's like wearing distorted glasses—everything seems warped, and you're constantly second-guessing yourself. This chapter is about clearing that fog so you can see the landscape of emotional and psychological abuse for what it truly is. It's not just about the bruises that show on the outside; it's about the scars that embed themselves deep within your psyche, unseen but profoundly felt.

2.1 Beyond Bruises: Emotional and Psychological Abuse Explained

Emotional and psychological abuse may not leave visible marks, but the wounds they inflict are just as real and often more difficult to heal. Unlike physical abuse, where the evidence can usually be seen and felt, the damage from emotional abuse lingers in the mind and spirit, hidden from the naked eye but painfully evident to the victim.

Defining Emotional Abuse

So, what exactly constitutes emotional abuse? It's a pattern of behavior that undermines an individual's mental health and sense of security. Emotional abusers systematically chip away at your confidence, your perceptions of reality, and your ability to react to your environment healthily. They deploy tactics such as invalidation, ridicule, and isolation—subtle tools that can be as damaging as any physical blow.

Imagine every time you express a concern, it's met with dismissal. "You're just too sensitive" or "You're overreacting" are phrases that might sound familiar. This is invalidation, where your feelings are routinely minimized or disregarded. Ridicule takes this further by dismissing and mocking your feelings, making you feel small and foolish. Isolation sneaks up on you as the abuser slowly, methodically cuts off your connections to others, making you increasingly dependent on them and their skewed perceptions of reality.

Impact on Self-Perception

The impact of such abuse on your self-esteem and self-worth is devastating. Over time, the constant criticism and gaslighting can distort how you see yourself. You may begin to believe that you are too sensitive, incapable, or unworthy of respect and love. This distorted self-perception is precisely what the abuser wants—it keeps you under their control, doubting yourself and your worth, and more importantly, questioning your ability to survive without them.

Legal Recognition and Rights

Thankfully, the legal system in many places is beginning to recognize the severe impact of emotional abuse. Various jurisdictions have laws that categorize psychological abuse as criminal, acknowledging that the harm it causes can be just as significant as physical harm. This recognition is crucial because it validates the experiences of victims and provides them with avenues to seek protection and justice. As a victim, understanding these legal rights can empower you to take steps towards escaping and healing from abusive situations. You have the right to feel safe and respected in your relationships—legally and personally.

Interactive Element: Reflection Section

To further explore and understand your own experiences, take a moment to reflect on these questions:

- Have there been times when you felt invalidated or ridiculed by someone close to you? How did it affect your feelings about yourself?
- Can you identify any relationships where you felt isolated from friends or family? What impact did this have on your relationship with the person isolating you?
- How aware are you of the legal protections against emotional abuse in your area?

Engaging with these questions can help you start to clear the fog of confusion that emotional abuse often creates, allowing you to see your experiences more clearly and assess them with a new perspective of understanding and acknowledgment.

This chapter aims to arm you with the knowledge and tools to recognize the signs of emotional and psychological abuse. By understanding what constitutes abuse, recognizing the behaviors involved, and knowing your rights, you can begin to take steps toward healing and reclaiming your life. Remember, the scars of emotional abuse, though invisible, are valid and significant. Your feelings are valid, your experiences are real, and you deserve a life free of abuse and full of respect and love. Remember, recognizing the abuse is the first step toward healing.

2.2 Identifying Toxic Behaviors in Everyday Life

Have you ever cringed at the ping of a text message, your stomach knotting up, not from anticipation but from dread? What might seem like just another day of navigating your social or work life is littered with subtle signs of toxicity that you've normalized. Recognizing these signs is like finally putting on the right prescription glasses after years of squinting through life.

Subtle signs of toxicity often manifest in ways that might not scream 'abuse' but are insidious enough to chip away at your peace of mind slowly. Let's talk about constant criticism first. Imagine sharing your daily happenings or ideas, only to be met with a barrage of why it's not good enough or how it could be better. It's like living with a personal critic who's perpetually unimpressed. Then, there's control over individual choices. Picture this: you're about to buy a new book or decide to join a gym, and your partner insists on picking the book or questions why you'd want to join that particular gym. It seems trivial, but over time, it's control masquerading as a concern. Lastly, manipulation of facts—where your reality is constantly questioned or rewritten (not to be confused with the overt gaslighting) to suit the narrative of another, leaving you doubting your memory or sanity.

Now, recognizing these patterns is crucial. Patterns might include the frequency of these behaviors or specific situations where they become more pronounced. For instance, does the criticism become harsher when you're in public, perhaps subtly under the guise of jokes? Or does the manipulation intensify when you make decisions that signify independence? Documenting these instances provides a tangible record that helps you see the frequency and context of these behaviors, which is especially useful when your experiences are being invalidated.

Ongoing toxic behaviors can profoundly affect all areas of your life. You might hesitate to share ideas at work, as an inner critic, influenced by someone else's negative voice, makes you doubt your abilities. Socially, you might withdraw out of fear of criticism or misunderstanding or constantly feel on edge, anticipating problems even in harmless situations. This constant state of hypervigilance is exhausting and can lead to anxiety, depression, or a persistent feeling of hopelessness.

Responding to these behaviors effectively requires a blend of assertiveness and boundary-setting. Assertive communication involves expressing your feelings and needs openly and honestly, without aggression. It's about saying, "When you dismiss my ideas regularly, I feel devalued. I need my thoughts to be considered with respect." Setting boundaries might mean deciding what you will no longer tolerate and communicating these limits. For example, "I appreciate constructive feedback, but constant negative remarks about my choices are not helpful, and I will not engage in discussions where this occurs." It's not about confrontation but about honoring your self-respect and emotional health.

Navigating through the fog of subtle toxic behaviors in your daily life isn't about finding fault in every interaction but about knowing how these interactions affect you. It's about recognizing patterns, understanding their impact, and responding in ways that preserve your well-being. Remember, the goal isn't to change the other person—a task likely beyond your control—but to change how you respond and what you're willing to accept in your interactions.

2.3 The Long-Term Effects of Narcissistic Abuse on Mental Health

Living with or escaping from a narcissistic relationship can feel like surviving a storm and then realizing the real challenge is rebuilding in the aftermath. The mental health conditions that emerge post-storm are not just remnants; they are profound indicators of the deep-seated trauma experienced. Among these, Post-Traumatic Stress Disorder (PTSD), anxiety, and depression are the most common shadows that follow survivors of narcissistic abuse. PTSD in this context isn't just about flashbacks or nightmares; it's about being in a constant state of hypervigilance, where even the slightest triggers can send you spiraling into anxiety. It's the persistent fear that the past might not be passed at all. Anxiety, meanwhile, might manifest in unrelenting worries about future relationships, self-worth, or safety, making relaxation and trust seem like languages you used to speak fluently but now barely understand. Depression often enters quietly, diminishing your energy and enthusiasm, making it difficult to remember a time when you felt hopeful or happy.

These conditions stitch a complex web, making day-to-day life a navigation through emotional landmines. Imagine planning a simple outing with friends but finding yourself frozen by the anxiety that you might inadvertently meet someone from your past. Or consider the effort it takes to start a new relationship when your baseline for normalcy has been recalibrated by years of manipulation. The fear of intimacy isn't just about fearing closeness; it's about protecting yourself from the devastation that might come if you trust again. It's a protective mechanism, yes, but it also isolates you, often reinforcing the very loneliness and sadness you're trying to escape.

Coping mechanisms adopted by survivors often start as survival strategies. However, when prolonged, tactics such as substance abuse or withdrawal from social activities can evolve into problematic behaviors. Substance abuse might begin as a way to numb the relentless anxiety or to quiet the memories that crowd your mind. Social withdrawal could start as a safety measure to avoid triggers, but over time, it can lead to isolation, which exacerbates feelings of depression and disconnection. It's like building a wall to protect yourself from a flood but finding you've also blocked the sunlight.

Healing from such deep psychological wounds requires a multifaceted approach. Therapy, especially trauma-informed therapy, can be a lighthouse for those navigating the foggy waters of recovery. It offers a space to voice your experiences and feelings without judgment, helping to dismantle the misplaced shame that often accompanies victims of narcissistic abuse. Cognitive-behavioral therapy (CBT), for instance, can be particularly effective in addressing PTSD by helping to reframe the negative thought patterns that are symptomatic of the disorder. Similarly, therapies that focus on mindfulness and emotional regulation can provide tools for managing anxiety, helping you learn to live in the present rather than being held hostage by past fears.

Beyond professional help, self-help strategies also play a crucial role in recovery. Establishing routine self-care practices—whether it's daily exercise, meditation, or engaging in hobbies that bring joy—can help rebuild the sense of normalcy and control that is often stripped away in abusive relationships. Journaling is another powerful tool, providing a private, reflective space to process emotions and track progress. It's like knitting together the narrative of your new life, one in which you are the author, not the character written by someone else's manipulation.

Incorporating these therapeutic approaches and self-help strategies doesn't erase the past. Still, it can significantly lighten the load of its impact, making the path forward a little more straightforward and hopeful. Remember, healing is not just about getting back to who you were before the narcissistic abuse; it's about discovering who you can be in its aftermath—stronger, wiser, and more whole than you might have ever imagined possible.

2.4 Why It's Hard to Spot: Subtle Abuse Tactics

Imagine you're in a maze; every turn feels right yet leads nowhere, and every sign seems helpful but leaves you more confused. This is often what navigating a relationship with a covert manipulator feels like. They employ insidious tactics woven into your daily interactions that spotting them can feel as elusive as finding a whisper in a whirlwind. Let's pull back the curtain on some of these tactics to spot them and understand their mechanics and effects.

Covert Manipulation

Covert manipulation is like the quiet hum of a refrigerator—it's always there, but you don't notice it until it stops. In the context of a relationship, this manipulation is often so embedded in interactions that it feels normal. Take gaslighting, for example, which we touched upon briefly before. It's more than just lying or denying—it's a series of actions to make you doubt your reality. Imagine expressing concern over something hurtful your partner said, only to be told, "That never happened," or, "You're imagining things." Over time, this persistent denial can lead you to distrust your memories and perceptions, a state of confusion that serves the manipulator's need to control.

These tactics aren't always overt or aggressive. They can be as subtle as a sigh, a smirk, or a sarcastic tone explained away as just joking. The abuser's denial of their manipulative intent, coupled with sporadic affirmations of love, keeps you second-guessing not just your perceptions but your judgment of the entire relationship. It's a psychological bind that keeps you tethered to the hope that the moments of kindness are more accurate than the manipulation, a hope that the abuser exploits time and again.

Isolation Tactics

Isolation is a crafty beast in the arsenal of an abuser. It starts small: a comment here about a friend's intentions, a slight about family members' influence. Over time, these comments can escalate into demands or emotional blackmail, pushing you to distance yourself from your support network. "If you loved me, you wouldn't need anyone else," they might say, framing it as a romantic ideal rather than a control tactic. The goal? To weaken your defenses by cutting you off from external perspectives and support, making you more dependent on the abuser for emotional sustenance and validation.

This isolation isn't just physical—it's emotional and intellectual, too. By monopolizing your attention and affection, the abuser can shape your reality, a particularly damaging effect. You might hesitate to share the good news with friends because you've been conditioned to believe they wouldn't understand or share in your joy. This erosion of external relationships deepens not only your isolation but also your reliance on the abuser, cementing your bond through dependency rather than genuine affection.

Cycles of Kindness and Cruelty

The push and pull of kindness and cruelty can create a confusing, emotional roller coaster. Think of it as the abuser throwing you off balance—when you're disoriented, you're easier to control. One day, you're the love of their life; the next, you can do nothing right. This unpredictability triggers a constant state of emotional turmoil, keeping you anxious and on edge. You might find yourself working tirelessly to recapture the abuser's affection, not realizing that this cycle is a calculated tactic to keep you invested in the relationship.

The cruelty often escalates when you show signs of strength or independence—it threatens their control. Conversely, the unexpected kindness that follows is not a genuine change of heart but a way to reel you back in, often when you're close to breaking away. This kindness acts as a period of respite and hope, a stark contrast to the cruelty that makes the good seem better and the bad more tolerable. It's a powerful manipulation that exploits your natural inclination for stability and love, turning your emotional world into a pendulum that swings at the whim of the abuser.

Normalization of Abuse

Normalization is perhaps the most insidious of the tactics because it transforms the unacceptable into the acceptable. Over time, the constant exposure to abuse desensitizes you to its presence—it becomes your new normal. The abuser might downplay their actions by comparing them to more severe forms of abuse, making you grateful for what you don't endure rather than aware of what you do. "At least I don't hit you," they might argue, framing their emotional or psychological abuse as not 'real' abuse.

This normalization extends beyond the relationship, influencing how others see the abuse, if they see it at all. Outsiders might view your relationship as passionate or tumultuous, not abusive. Even when you know something is wrong, the validation from others that "it's not that bad" can persuade you to minimize your own experiences. This societal echo of the abuser's perspective serves to entrench the abuse further, making it harder to recognize and even harder to escape.

Understanding these tactics isn't just about spotting them; it's about seeing through them. It's about recognizing the patterns and intentions behind the actions, which can empower you to reclaim your perceptions, relationships, and life. Remember, the subtlety of these tactics makes them powerful, but your awareness and actions can dismantle that power, one truth at a time.

2.5 Trauma Bonding: Why You Feel Stuck

Imagine, if you will, that you're glued to a chair. You can see the dangers looming; you feel the discomfort, yet despite every logical part of you screaming to get up and move, something keeps you seated. That 'something' is akin to trauma bonding, a concept that's as complex as it is devastating. Trauma bonding forms under conditions where intermittent reinforcement of reward and punishment creates powerful emotional bonds that resist change. In simpler terms, it's the stick-and-carrot approach but with high-stakes emotional manipulation.

Trauma bonding is often formed in relationships characterized by high intensity, unpredictability, a constant fear of danger, or where one person feels they have no better options. The bonds are forged through cycles of abuse followed by kindness. When an abuser throws in an unexpected kindness or an apology after a cycle of cruelty, it triggers a profound sense of relief and gratitude in the victim. This intermittent reinforcement feeds a hope for resolution, a belief in change, which paradoxically binds the victim closer to their abuser.

Signs that a trauma bond has formed can be subtle or overt. You might find yourself defending the abuser to friends and family, rationalizing their behavior, and focusing on the 'good times.' You might feel an overwhelming loyalty to them, even when you logically understand the relationship is harmful. Another significant sign is feeling unable to leave the relationship despite repeated harm. This isn't just about loving someone; it's about feeling psychologically tethered to them, where thoughts of leaving trigger immense anxiety and fears of not just being alone but of being unable to cope alone.

The psychological effects of trauma bonding can be profound and long-lasting. The bond itself is characterized by a deep-rooted dependency on the abuser, not just emotionally but often financially or socially. It creates persistent doubt in one's ability to function independently and fosters a misplaced loyalty or responsibility to the abuser, often at significant cost to one's mental health. Feelings of worthlessness, helplessness, or being trapped are not uncommon, nor is a persistent state of fear or walking on eggshells.

Breaking a trauma bond is challenging and usually requires multiple strategies. The first step is recognizing the bond and its impact on your life and self. It's akin to realizing the chair you're glued to is on fire. Recognition alone can be painful, often bringing up shame or guilt, but it's crucial. This is where professional help can be invaluable. Therapists, particularly those experienced in dealing with trauma and abuse, can offer not just insight but practical strategies to start loosening the glue binding you to the chair.

Support networks play a critical role, too. Reconnecting with friends and family can provide not just emotional support but a reality check on the dynamics of the abusive relationship. Often, isolation is a tactic used by abusers to strengthen trauma bonds, and rebuilding your social network can counteract this. Support groups can also provide solace and strength, whether online or in person. Hearing others' stories of similar experiences can validate your feelings and experiences, reducing the shame and isolation that often accompanies trauma bonds.

Practical steps to breaking the bond include setting physical and emotional boundaries or, in some cases, cutting off contact with the abuser. This might involve changing phone numbers, blocking them on social media, or even moving to a new location. Financial independence is crucial, too; start creating a financial exit plan that allows you to stand on your own two feet. This means opening a separate bank account, seeking employment, or saving quietly.

Recognizing and breaking a trauma bond demands courage, support, and often professional guidance. Still, it's a path that leads out of the maze of manipulation and back to a life where you can stand up from the chair and walk away into a healthier, autonomous future. Remember, the journey to recovery is not just about escaping the bond but about rediscovering and reclaiming your sense of self outside of it.

2.6 Breaking Down Denial: Facing the Reality of Abuse

Denial is a thick, often impenetrable curtain that shields us from truths too painful to accept. It's the "No, it can't be" that echoes in our minds when faced with the stark reality of abuse. For victims, the reasons for denial are as complex as they are compelling. Fear stands tall among these reasons—it's the fear of the consequences of acknowledging the abuse, whether it involves personal safety, financial security, or the daunting prospect of starting over. Then there's the shame, a corrosive emotion that whispers lies about one's worthiness and clouds judgment. It tells you it's your fault or that acknowledging the abuse is an admission of weakness. Coupled with a lack of knowledge about what constitutes abuse, incredibly emotional and psychological, these factors create a potent cocktail that makes denial a preferred refuge to facing the grim realities.

The steps to acknowledgment are akin to walking through a dense fog, where each step reveals more of the path ahead. The first step is often the hardest: recognizing the signs of abuse. This involves educating yourself about what abuse looks like—not just the overt types but the subtle, insidious kinds that leave no bruises but deep emotional scars. Next, allowing yourself to feel the emotions that come with this recognition is crucial—anger, grief, disbelief. These feelings are not just expected but essential to your healing process.

Once you've begun to face the reality of your situation, seeking validation can be incredibly empowering. This is where a supportive network comes into play. Talking to friends, family, or a professional who affirms your experiences can be a powerful antidote to the isolation and self-doubt that abuse engenders. It's not just about confirming that the abuse occurred; it's about reaffirming your worth, your right to safety and happiness, and your strength in facing these truths.

Moving from victim to survivor is not just a change in terminology; it's a profound shift in mindset and self-perception. It involves redefining your identity beyond the abuse, recognizing your inherent strength, and reclaiming your autonomy. Emotional strategies like affirmations—simple statements like "I am worthy of respect" or "I deserve safety and love"—can fortify this transition. Mentally, it requires a deliberate focus on the future, where you are not defined by what happened to you but by how you've grown from it.

This phase of your healing journey is about building, or rebuilding, a life that reflects your worth and aspirations. It's a testament to your resilience and a foundation for a future where abuse has no place. Remember, acknowledging abuse is not just about ending a cycle of violence; it's about beginning a cycle of recovery and empowerment, where you step into the light of truth and refuse to go back into the shadows.

As we wrap up this chapter, it's essential to reflect on the journey of breaking through denial to face the harsh truths of abuse. From understanding the reasons behind denial to taking the critical steps toward acknowledgment, the path is fraught with challenges and opportunities for profound personal growth. Seeking validation and shifting from a victim to a survivor mindset are not just steps in recovery; they are strides toward reclaiming your life. As you go on, remember that abuse is powerful darkness, but your ability to find the light is unbeatable. The next chapter will build on these foundations, exploring practical strategies and tools to fortify your journey from acknowledgment to empowerment, ensuring that each step is rooted in strength, clarity, and an unwavering commitment to your well-being.

Chapter 3
Strategies for Emotional Protection

Imagine you're navigating a rocky path, uneven and unpredictable. Suddenly, it starts to rain, not just a drizzle but a torrential downpour. You're soaked and cold, and the path becomes even more treacherous. But then, you remember—you've packed a raincoat and an umbrella. Armed with these, the route isn't necessarily more accessible, but you feel protected, secure, and ready to continue your journey. This is what emotional self-defense is all about: equipping yourself with tools and strategies to protect against the storms of narcissistic abuse, ensuring you can continue forward, no matter the weather.

3.1 Emotional Self-Defense: Effective Coping Mechanisms

Navigating life with a narcissist can sometimes feel like being in a perpetual storm. Developing robust emotional self-defense mechanisms is the key to surviving and thriving in this environment. It's about recognizing when it's starting to 'rain' and knowing how to stay dry.

Identify Triggers

First, let's talk about identifying your emotional triggers. These are specific actions or words that, when expressed by the narcissist, deeply affect your emotional state. It might be a particular tone of voice, a dismissive gesture, or even a specific time of day when past arguments typically occurred. Recognizing these triggers is like mapping the clouds before the storm—they give you a heads-up that you might need to prepare for emotional turbulence.

Understanding your triggers can help you manage your responses in a way that maintains your emotional equilibrium. For example, suppose you know that being criticized in public triggers you. In that case, you can prepare by rehearsing calm responses or deciding in advance to remove yourself from the situation temporarily. This preemptive approach doesn't just reduce the emotional impact at the moment; it also helps build your resilience over time.

Developing Emotional Resilience

Building emotional resilience is akin to strengthening your core muscles; it helps you maintain balance, no matter how uneven the ground gets. Techniques like mindfulness and emotional regulation are your exercises here. Mindfulness, which involves staying present and fully engaging with the here and now, can help you recognize the onset of an emotional reaction without immediately succumbing to it. It's like noticing the wind picking up and zipping up your jacket.

Emotional regulation techniques, such as deep breathing or grounding exercises, can help manage your emotional reactions once they're triggered. These are your emotional raincoat and boots, keeping you dry and steady. By practicing these techniques regularly, not just when you're triggered, you build up your emotional resilience, making it easier to handle future 'storms.'

Creating Emotional Buffers

Emotional buffers are activities or relationships that provide a protective barrier against narcissistic abuse. These can be hobbies, support groups, or therapeutic practices that help reinforce your sense of self and maintain your emotional health. Think of them as the scenic shelters you might find along your path—places to rest and rejuvenate.

Engaging in activities you love and reminding yourself of your worth can be incredibly protective. Whether painting, hiking, or playing music, these activities break you from the emotional turbulence and remind you of your identity beyond the relationship. Support groups or therapy can also act as buffers, providing empathy and understanding from others who know what walking in your shoes is like.

Emergency Emotional Safety Plans

Finally, having an emergency emotional safety plan in place is crucial. This is your evacuation route when the emotional weather turns severe. Such a plan might include a list of contacts—friends, family, or a therapist—who can offer immediate support, a physical place where you feel safe, and activities that can help calm and center you, like breathing exercises or a comforting playlist.

Creating this plan involves thinking about what you need during a crisis and organizing these resources ahead of time. For instance, if physical exercise helps calm your mind, your safety plan might include a quick walk or a yoga session. Having this plan written down, perhaps in a journal or on your phone, ensures that you don't have to think; you can just act, following the steps you've laid out to safeguard your emotional well-being.

Incorporating these strategies into your daily life doesn't just help you cope with the challenges of living with or moving beyond a narcissistic relationship; they empower you to lead a happier, more balanced life. They're not just about weathering storms but about enjoying the journey, rain or shine.

3.2 Mastering Detachment: Techniques for Emotional Disengagement

Imagine you're at a bustling street fair, surrounded by noise, colors, and crowds. Now, picture yourself putting on a pair of noise-canceling headphones. Suddenly, the chaos dims, and while you're still aware of the environment, you're not overwhelmed. This is what emotional detachment can feel like when dealing with a narcissist. It's not about ignoring the presence or denying the significance of the narcissist in your life; it's about adjusting your settings to manage better the impact they have on your emotional landscape.

Understanding Detachment

Firstly, let's clarify what emotional detachment means in the context of interacting with a narcissist. It's a conscious effort to maintain your emotional boundaries by not allowing yourself to be swept up in the narcissist's dramas or manipulated by their emotional outbursts. It's essential because, without this detachment, you may find yourself constantly on an emotional rollercoaster, controlled by someone else's dysfunctional behaviors. Detachment helps you to conserve your emotional energy and prioritize your mental health.

The process of detachment is akin to setting an emotional thermostat. Just as you wouldn't leave your windows open in a blizzard, you shouldn't expose your emotional well-being to the whims of a narcissist. It means noticing when someone is trying to manipulate your emotions and deciding not to overreact.

Practical Steps to Detachment

Detaching from a narcissist requires a mix of awareness, practice, and resilience. Start by identifying the situations where you feel most emotionally vulnerable. These are your high-risk times for becoming entangled in the narcissist's emotional manipulations. Once you've identified these situations, you can practice maintaining your calm. This involves deep breathing exercises, mentally stepping back to observe the situation as if you were a third party, or even excusing yourself from the environment.

Keeping your emotional reactions private is another crucial step in detachment. The less the narcissist knows about how they affect you, the less they can tailor their manipulations to push your buttons. This doesn't mean shutting down your emotions; instead, it means choosing to express them in a safe, controlled environment, perhaps with a therapist or trusted friend, rather than in the presence of the narcissist.

Maintaining Personal Boundaries

Firm personal boundaries are the foundation of effective emotional detachment. These rules and limits you set for yourself in interactions with others help you manage how much you engage emotionally and how much of your personal life you share. Enforcing these boundaries consistently can be challenging, mainly if the narcissist in your life is used to having them disregarded. However, you reinforce your right to emotional autonomy whenever you assert your boundaries.

Setting these boundaries might include deciding not to respond to attempts to bait you into arguments or emotional scenes. It might mean limiting the topics you are willing to discuss or the time you spend together. The key is consistency; the more consistently you enforce your boundaries, the stronger they become.

Role of Detachment in Healing

Emotional detachment plays a critical role in the healing process. By learning to detach from the narcissist's emotional world, you reclaim control over your own. This can be incredibly empowering, particularly if you've been entangled in their emotional games for a long time. Detachment allows you to step back and assess the relationship more objectively, which is often the first step towards making healthy changes, whether that means deepening your boundaries within the relationship or, if necessary, considering more significant changes, such as ending the relationship.

Moreover, detachment helps reduce the impact of the narcissist's behavior on your day-to-day emotional state. It enables you to break the cycle of emotional reaction and retaliation, which not only preserves your mental health but can also lead to a more peaceful life. As you practice detachment, you can better enjoy your life, engage more fully with others, and pursue your personal goals without the constant distraction of emotional turbulence.

By mastering the techniques of emotional detachment, you equip yourself with a vital tool not just for navigating relationships with narcissists but for enhancing your overall emotional well-being. It's about learning to stay centered in your own emotional experience and not getting pulled into someone else's chaos, no matter how close they are. This skill, once developed, can serve you in many areas of life, ensuring that your emotional energy goes where it truly belongs—to your own life and aspirations.

3.3 Responding to Narcissistic Rage: A Tactical Guide

When the storm of narcissistic rage shatters the calm of your day, it can feel like you're suddenly thrust onto a stage without a script, the spotlight glaring down relentlessly. Understanding this tempestuous behavior and arming yourself with strategies to navigate it is akin to finding that script tucked away in your back pocket, giving you lines that calm the storm or sidestep it altogether.

Narcissistic rage can be sparked by what might seem like a trivial matter to others but feels like a monumental threat to the narcissist's ego. It's a dramatic reaction to a perceived slight, criticism, or disagreement, and recognizing the early signs of this rage is crucial. These signs might include a noticeable shift in tone, quickening speech, or even subtle changes in body language, such as clenching fists or stiffening posture. The air might feel charged, a silent alarm that, if you've come to know, signals the need to tread carefully.

In these moments, de-escalation becomes your most valuable tactic. This isn't about placating or appeasing but rather about bringing the temperature down and protecting both of you from the consequences of an outburst. Effective de-escalation techniques include maintaining a calm and even tone, using non-confrontational language, and physically positioning yourself in a non-threatening way—this means no crossed arms, direct confrontational stances, or intense eye contact. Phrases that can help might include "I see you're upset, and that's not my intention" or "Let's talk about this when we're both calm." Conversely, avoid accusatory or inflammatory language and resist the urge to defend yourself aggressively, which can further escalate the situation.

Safety planning is an essential aspect of dealing with narcissistic rage. The situation might not cool down despite your best de-escalation efforts. Knowing when and how to remove yourself from the problem is crucial. Have a pre-planned exit strategy for each environment where you might encounter rage. This might mean knowing which room you can go to lock the door, having a bag packed if you need to leave suddenly, or even having a code word with a friend or family member that means "come help" or "call me."

Accessing professional help and legal protection is crucial if the rage escalates to threats or physical abuse. Familiarize yourself with local resources like hotlines, shelters, and legal advice for domestic situations. Reporting threats and abuse might feel daunting, but legal professionals and law enforcement train to handle such situations with confidentiality and tact. Remember, prioritizing your safety is not just a right; it's a necessity.

Navigating through narcissistic rage requires a blend of awareness, preparedness, and resilience. By recognizing the signs, employing de-escalation techniques, ensuring your safety, and knowing how to access professional and legal resources, you can survive these challenging encounters and manage them with strength and assurance. Remember, you're not responsible for the narcissist's emotions or reactions, but you are responsible for your safety and well-being. Equip yourself with knowledge and strategies, and take back control over your emotional environment.

3.4 The Art of Grey Rock: Becoming Emotionally Uninteresting

Imagine you're at a party, and there's that one person who thrives on drama and attention. Now, think about how you might make yourself less interesting to them. You might talk about mundane things like the weather or how you organize your sock drawer. That's essentially what the Grey Rock Method is about—it's a strategy for interacting with narcissists by making yourself as dull and unengaging as possible. Why? Because narcissists thrive on the emotional responses of others, it's their version of applause. By denying them this, you become less appealing and less of a target for their manipulations.

The Grey Rock Method is beneficial because it focuses on controlling your responses to the narcissist's attempts to provoke you. It's not about changing them; it's about changing how you interact with them. When you're as emotionally expressive as a grey rock, there's nothing for the narcissist to exploit. But how do you implement this in fundamental interactions? It starts with mastering the art of non-engagement. This means keeping conversations superficial and brief. If a narcissist is trying to bait you into an argument or emotional reaction, your responses should be as neutral and uninteresting as possible. Think of phrases like "Hmm," "I see," or

"That's interesting." Keep your tone even and your facial expressions minimal.

Practicing this method can be more challenging than it sounds, especially if you're naturally expressive or if the narcissist knows how to push your buttons. One effective strategy is to prepare a mental list of bland, non-committal responses before interacting with them. Rehearse these responses so that you can use them automatically, reducing the risk of slipping into more engaging dialogue. Another tip is to visualize yourself as an actor playing the role of the most boring character imaginable. This tip will create psychological distance between your true feelings and outward demeanor.

Challenges and Considerations

While the Grey Rock Method can be a powerful tool for dealing with narcissists, it's not without its challenges. One of the biggest is maintaining consistency, especially when faced with aggressive or provocative behavior. It's natural to want to defend yourself or to react emotionally. However, doing so can draw you back into the engagement cycle you're trying to break. It can be helpful to remember that the goal of grey rocking is protection, not confrontation. Reminding yourself of this purpose can help you stay focused on your strategy, even when provoked.

Another consideration is the emotional impact of consistently dampening your reactions, which can feel unnatural and even stressful, particularly over extended periods. It's essential to find healthy outlets for your emotions outside of your interactions with the narcissist. Engage in activities that allow you to express yourself fully, whether that's through creative pursuits, exercise, or discussions with supportive friends or family. This engagement helps prevent the build-up of suppressed emotions, which can be damaging to your mental health.

Long-term Effects

Using the Grey Rock Method can significantly affect your relationships and emotional health. On the positive side, it can reduce conflict and emotional turmoil. As the narcissist receives fewer emotional reactions from you, they may find less gratification in trying to provoke you and turn their attention elsewhere, creating a more peaceful life and giving you more excellent emotional stability.

However, excessive grey rocking might also lead to feelings of isolation or detachment in other relationships. Monitoring how this strategy affects your overall ability to connect and engage with others is crucial. Make sure to balance your interactions with the narcissist with plenty of genuine, fulfilling emotional interactions with others.

Regular self-care is vital to maintaining emotional health using the Grey Rock Method. Ensure you have a robust support system, and consider working with a therapist who can help you navigate the complexities of your relationship with the narcissist. They can provide you with tools to implement grey rocking more effectively and handle the emotional strain it can cause.

Incorporating the Grey Rock Method into your interactions with a narcissist can be like putting up an emotional shield. It protects you from their attempts to manipulate and destabilize your emotional world. Any defensive strategy requires practice, consistency, and a clear understanding of when and how to use it effectively. Remember, the ultimate goal is safeguarding your emotional well-being, allowing you to lead a more peaceful and controlled life despite ongoing challenges.

3.5 Protecting Your Mental Space: Tips and Tools

Imagine your mind as a private garden. What grows there is primarily determined by the seeds you plant and your attention to nurturing your space. In this garden, negative thoughts or external stressors are like weeds. They can sprout up seemingly out of nowhere and, if not managed, might overtake the vibrant, healthy plants you've worked so hard to cultivate. In the context of dealing with narcissistic abuse, safeguarding this mental space becomes not just beneficial but necessary for your emotional well-being and personal growth. Here, we'll explore how to foster a positive mental environment, use affirmations effectively, harness the calming power of mindfulness and meditation, and set meaningful emotional and mental health goals.

Cultivating a Positive Mental Environment

The quality of your mental environment can significantly influence how you perceive and react to the world around you. Creating and maintaining a positive mental space starts with intentional practices such as engaging in positive self-talk and limiting your exposure to negativity, which means setting boundaries around how much negative news you consume or distancing yourself from toxic relationships that drain your emotional energy.

Positive self-talk is particularly powerful. It involves consciously shifting your internal dialogue to be more encouraging and affirming. For instance, instead of telling yourself, "I can't handle this," you might say, "I have handled difficult situations before, and I can work through this too." This shift doesn't mean ignoring your challenges but rather framing them in a way that affirms your ability to cope and thrive.

The spaces you frequent also influence your mental state. Creating a physical environment that reflects calmness and positivity can internally reinforce a sense of peace and order. Organizing your living space to reduce clutter, decorating with colors and items that bring you joy, or establishing a special nook to relax and recharge are options to reinforce this sense.

Use of Affirmations

Affirmations are positive statements that can help combat the often ingrained negative messaging received from a narcissist. These statements are most effective when they are personal, positive, present tense, and precise. For example, an affirmation like "I am worthy of respect and love" directly counters the feelings of worthlessness that narcissistic abuse might foster.

To incorporate affirmations into your daily routine, write them on Post-it notes and place them where you'll see them throughout the day, like on your bathroom mirror or the refrigerator. Saying these affirmations out loud, especially at the start and end of your day, can reinforce their power, embedding these positive beliefs deeper into your subconscious.

Mindfulness and Meditation

Mindfulness and meditation are like personal tune-ups for your brain. They help clear away mental clutter, allowing you to maintain focus and calm in chaos. Mindfulness involves staying present and fully engaged with the here and now. It can be practiced at any moment, whether washing dishes, walking, or listening to music. The key is to absorb the present activity without judgment or distraction fully.

Meditation, on the other hand, often involves setting aside time to focus inward, whether it's through guided imagery, breathing exercises, or silent contemplation. For those new to meditation, starting with just a few minutes daily can be beneficial. Numerous apps and online resources offer guided meditations to enhance calm and focus.

Setting Emotional and Mental Goals

Setting regular emotional and mental health goals is a proactive way to ensure your well-being is not lost in daily responsibilities. These goals can be as simple as achieving a certain level of tranquility each day or as specific as dedicating weekly time to engaging in activities that boost your mental health.

Tracking your progress can be both motivating and insightful. It allows you to see patterns in your emotional well-being that you might otherwise miss and provides a tangible measure of your personal growth. You might use reflection on your emotional state at the end of each day or a digital app to rate your mood and note activities that increase your well-being.

Incorporating these strategies into your life not only enhances your ability to deal with the impacts of narcissistic abuse but also builds a foundation for long-term emotional resilience and happiness. By actively cultivating a positive mental environment, using affirmations to reinforce your self-worth, practicing mindfulness to maintain mental clarity, and setting specific emotional and mental health goals, you empower yourself to lead a more prosperous, more balanced life. Through these practices, you ensure that your mental garden flourishes, making it a sanctuary of peace and positivity, resilient against the weeds of negativity and stress.

3.6 Self-Validation Techniques to Counter Doubt and Gaslighting

Imagine you're painting a picture, but every stroke you make is questioned or criticized by someone peering over your shoulder. This individual says your blues are too dull, and your perspective is wrong. After a while, you might start to believe them, doubting your artistic choices, perhaps even your ability to paint. Constant exposure to gaslighting and doubt shakes the foundation of your confidence, making you question your perceptions and memories. Self-validation is taking back the paintbrush and trusting in your ability to create your picture, your reality.

Understanding Self-Validation

Self-validation is affirming your emotions, thoughts, and experiences, regardless of external input. It's essential in countering the effects of gaslighting, where a narcissist might attempt to overwrite your reality with their own to maintain control. By validating yourself, you reinforce your trust in your perceptions and feelings, which is crucial in keeping your mental health and emotional independence.

Imagine self-validation as building a fort around your sense of self. Each affirmation is a brick; each act of trust in your feelings is a reinforcement. This fort protects you from external doubts and manipulations, making you feel secure within your perceptions.

It's not about convincing yourself that you're always right but rather about trusting yourself enough to know when something feels off, or someone's actions are harmful, regardless of their explanations or excuses.

Techniques for Self-Validation

One powerful technique for self-validation is journaling. Writing down your thoughts and feelings helps solidify them. It acts as a mirror reflecting your internal world, unaffected by the distortions someone else might try to impose. When you journal, focus on how events made you feel rather than just the events themselves. This practice reinforces that your emotional responses are valid and provides a documented record that you can look back on, which can be incredibly helpful in moments of doubt.

Seeking external affirmations from trusted individuals can also bolster your self-validation. External affirmations do not rely solely on others to define your reality but instead use their perspectives to support or affirm your own. Choose people who have a history of understanding and helping you and are not connected to the narcissist. Their affirmation can act as a counterbalance to gaslighting, reminding you that your perceptions are not only valid but shared by others.

Another effective self-validation strategy is using logic to dispute gaslighting claims. Using logic involves critically assessing the narcissist's arguments and looking for inconsistencies or manipulations. For example, if a narcissist claims an event didn't happen, yet you have a text or a witness who can confirm it did, this evidence can help reaffirm your version of reality.

Role of Professional Help

In situations where gaslighting has severely eroded your confidence in your perceptions and memories, professional help can be invaluable. Therapists, especially those experienced in dealing with narcissistic abuse, can provide a safe space to explore and validate your experiences. They can help you develop tools for self-validation, offer objective insights into your interactions, and support you in rebuilding your trust in yourself. Therapy can be a sanctuary where your voice is heard and believed, helping you reconstruct your self-esteem on a foundation of validated, personal truth.

Community and Support Networks

Lastly, engaging with community and support networks can significantly enhance your self-validation efforts. Support groups, both online and in-person, connect you with others who have similar experiences. These communities can provide a collective validation that is incredibly powerful against the isolating effects of gaslighting. They remind you that you are not alone, that your experiences are real, and that others share your struggles and triumphs.

Participating in these communities can also strengthen your ability to trust your perceptions. Hearing others articulate similar feelings or experiences can confirm your reality, reinforcing that you are not the outlier the narcissist might have you believe. These networks provide both validation and collective wisdom on coping strategies, further empowering you to trust and validate your experiences.

By incorporating these self-validation techniques into your life, you not only counter the effects of doubt and gaslighting but also build a stronger, more resilient sense of self. Self-validation is a shield foundation, protecting you from external manipulations and supporting your personal growth and autonomy. Once honed, it can be used in every aspect of your life, ensuring that the strokes are all your own when you paint your picture.

As this chapter closes, remember that the self-validation journey is personal and empowering. It's about reclaiming your narrative, trusting your inner self, and affirming your right to your emotions and experiences. As we move forward, we will explore further strategies to not just cope with narcissistic abuse but thrive despite it, ensuring each step you take is grounded in confidence and self-belief.

Chapter 4
Setting and Enforcing Boundaries

Imagine you're at a bustling street market, surrounded by people, noise, and a dizzying array of smells. Everyone wants something from you—vendors calling out, trying to call you to their stalls. Now, imagine you have a clear, comfortable bubble around you. It's invisible but keeps you at a comfortable distance, allowing you to interact on your terms. This bubble? It's your boundary, and just like in that crowded market, it helps you navigate through life's chaos, especially when dealing with a narcissist.

4.1 Boundary Basics: Defining and Establishing Your Limits

Understanding the Concept of Boundaries

Boundaries are your limits that define how you would like to be treated; they are guidelines that inform others about how they can behave around you. These boundaries can be emotional, physical, or even digital. Emotional boundaries relate to your feelings and how much energy you allow yourself to absorb from others. Physical boundaries pertain to your personal space and physical touch. Digital boundaries, meanwhile, govern your engagement with technology and social media—what you share, when you are available, and how people can interact with you online.

Especially in relationships involving narcissists, boundaries are less about building walls and more about drawing lines in the sand. Without these lines, a narcissist may claim too much of your emotional beachfront property, leaving you with little room to build your sandcastles of self-esteem and personal space.

Steps to Establish Boundaries

Establishing boundaries with a narcissist is like setting up a fence in your backyard; it's about creating a clear demarcation point where your property begins and ends. Firstly, identify what you are comfortable with. How often are you willing to communicate, and how do you expect to be treated in conversations? Here's a simple exercise: list instances from past interactions that made you uncomfortable or overstepped. Reflect on these and determine what limit, if upheld, would have prevented these feelings.

Once you've identified these limits, articulate them clearly. You can start small. For instance, if uninterrupted personal time is essential, you might set a boundary by saying, "I value our conversations, but I need the hour after dinner as quiet time for myself." It's direct, simple, and informs the other person of your needs and expectations without being confronted.

Role of Self-Awareness

Being self-aware is like being the captain of your ship; you need to know where your boat leaks, what cargo it carries, and when it sails best. In the context of setting boundaries, this means knowing your emotional triggers, understanding your values, and recognizing your limits. Your personality and experiences deeply influence these elements. For instance, if you value loyalty, a lack of empathy and prioritizing their needs and desires are significant triggers. Recognizing this will help you set boundaries around behaviors that demonstrate commitment and reliability.

Setting Realistic Boundaries

The key to setting boundaries that work is ensuring they are realistic and enforceable. It's like planting a garden; you wouldn't plant tropical flowers in a cold climate. Similarly, setting a boundary that you know you cannot enforce or that is constantly ignored might need reevaluation. Consider your environment—both personal and social. A boundary like expecting no calls after 8 PM might be reasonable with friends but not with family members with whom you have a different dynamic.

Communicate these boundaries clearly and consistently. It's not enough to set a boundary; you must enforce it. This might mean reminding others of your boundaries when they forget or distancing yourself from situations where your limits are not respected. Like training vines to climb a trellis, it takes patience and persistence to guide the growth in your desired direction.

In this section, we have navigated the foundational aspects of setting boundaries. Understanding and establishing these limits is crucial, particularly in relationships fraught with the complexities of narcissism. As you continue to fortify your boundaries, remember that each step is a step towards a healthier, more balanced interaction with those around you.

4.2 Practical Scenarios: Handling Boundary Violations

Imagine you're enjoying a peaceful afternoon in your garden, sipping tea and relishing the solitude, when suddenly, a soccer ball comes flying over the fence, disrupting your tranquility. This invasion, albeit small, is similar to when someone crosses your boundaries—it's unexpected, jarring, and can leave you feeling violated. Recognizing when your limits have been breached and responding to these violations is crucial. Let's explore how to identify and effectively handle these moments to maintain peace and assert your needs.

When a boundary is crossed, it might not always come with a physical intrusion like a soccer ball in your sanctuary. More often, it's subtle—a friend repeatedly calling late at night despite your request for no calls after a particular hour or a co-worker continually borrowing your items without asking. These actions might stir up feelings of irritation, anger, or betrayal. Recognizing these feelings is your first cue that a boundary has been crossed. It's essential to listen to these emotional signals; they are your internal defense system alerting you to potential oversteps.

Once you've recognized a violation, the next step is to respond effectively. This isn't about retaliation but reasserting your boundaries to prevent future breaches. Assertive communication is your tool here. It involves expressing your feelings clearly and respectfully without being aggressive. For instance, if a friend has called late again, you might say, "I noticed you called after 9 PM a few times this week. I must stick to my routine, so please respect my request not to receive calls after this time." This statement is direct and expresses your needs without blaming or shaming the other person.

In situations where the boundary-pusher might react defensively, it's helpful to maintain a calm demeanor and use "I" statements. These phrases focus on your feelings rather than accusing the other person, which can help keep the conversation from escalating. Remember, the goal is to be heard and respected, not to win an argument.

Not every boundary violation is a sign of disrespect; sometimes, people forget or test limits unconsciously. These moments can be learning opportunities. Reflect on each incident and consider whether your boundary was communicated from the start. The boundary may have been too rigid or unrealistic in specific contexts. Use these reflections to adjust your boundaries, ensuring they are clear and reasonable. This might mean having a follow-up conversation to clarify your expectations or changing your behavior to reinforce these limits.

Preventive measures are also essential in managing boundaries. Setting clear, consistent precedents early in any relationship—personal or professional—helps establish a mutual understanding of respect and consideration. For example, proactively informing new acquaintances of your communication preferences can prevent future misunderstandings and violations. Clear communication about your boundaries sets the tone for your interactions and teaches others how to engage with you respectfully from the outset.

You can maintain your personal space and dignity by recognizing when your boundaries have been crossed, responding assertively, learning from these violations, and taking preventive steps. Each of these steps reinforces the importance of your needs and well-being, ensuring that your garden remains a sanctuary, undisturbed by unwanted intrusions.

4.3 Communicating Boundaries to a Narcissist

Talking about setting boundaries with a narcissist can sometimes feel like explaining quantum physics to your pet cat. You might lay out your best, most logical points, but all you get in return is a blank stare or an unexpected swipe. Narcissists, with their particular blend of needing dominance and lacking empathy, often react to boundaries with everything from cold denial to outright aggression. It's not just that they don't like being told no; boundaries directly challenge their worldview, where they prefer to operate without constraints, especially in their behavior towards others.

Let's tackle this tricky scenario. Imagine you're setting a boundary about not wanting to discuss your job during family dinners. A simple and reasonable request, right? However, when dealing with a narcissist, this straightforward communication can trigger a disproportionate reaction. They might accuse you of keeping secrets or being overly sensitive, turning a simple boundary into a personal critique. In these moments, it's crucial to use clear and non-confrontational language. Phrases like "I feel overwhelmed discussing work at dinner and would prefer to focus on enjoying our meal together" center your feelings rather than their behavior, making it harder for the narcissist to argue without blatantly disregarding your feelings.

Staying calm and consistent is your armor here. Narcissists feed on emotional reactions; your upset is their victory. By maintaining a quiet demeanor, you starve them of the response they seek, which can de-escalate the situation. Consistency is your sword.

Each time the boundary is tested, your calm response reinforces that this isn't a one-time rule but a standard. Over time, this consistency can condition a level of respect for your boundaries, even from someone as typically resistant as a narcissist. It's not about changing their personality but modifying their expectations about what behavior they will tolerate.

Dealing with the backlash is where things get prickly. When a boundary is set, some narcissists might retaliate with everything from silent treatment to verbal assaults. This backlash is a test, a storm you need to weather. Stick to your assertions. A gentle but firm reminder of your boundaries is necessary if you've asked not to discuss work at dinner and the topic is brought up. "I understand you're interested, but like I mentioned, I'm not comfortable discussing work right now. Let's talk about our plans for the weekend instead." This pivot not only reinforces your boundary but also offers an alternative, keeping the interaction from coming to a complete stop.

Navigating these interactions requires a blend of firmness and flexibility, a dance where you hold your ground without stepping on too many toes. It's nuanced, sometimes exhausting, but incredibly necessary. By setting and maintaining clear boundaries, you teach the narcissist how to engage with you in a way that respects your space and emotional well-being. This doesn't just improve your interactions; it fundamentally alters the dynamic, shifting it from subjugation to mutual respect, at least in respecting boundaries. Remember, while you can't control their reactions, you can control your boundaries and how steadfastly you uphold them. This control is your right; exercising it is a testament to your strength and self-respect. Keep calm, stay consistent, and let your boundaries be known clearly and unapologetically. In doing so, you carve out a space where your needs are acknowledged, and you can breathe easier, even in the most challenging relationships.

No soldier goes into battle without backup, and in the skirmishes of boundary-setting, your support system is your battalion. Whether it's friends who respect your limits, family who cheers on your assertiveness, or a therapist who provides a professional perspective, these allies can bolster your resolve. They offer a sounding board for your frustrations, advice for your uncertainties, and sometimes, just the reassurance that you're on the right path. After a challenging interaction about boundaries, a quick chat with a supportive friend can remind you that you're not overreacting but simply respecting yourself. This validation is often the boost needed to stand firm in your decisions.

In navigating the pushback that inevitably comes with setting boundaries, especially with a narcissist, remember that each challenge is both a test and a confirmation. It tests your commitment to your rules and confirms their necessity. So, as you firm up your boundaries, each effort to maintain them, each strategy employed, and each support enlisted doesn't just protect your garden—it helps it flourish. As you get better at this, you'll notice something incredible: you are becoming proficient at safeguarding your space and teaching others how to respect it, one boundary at a time.

Unmask Narcissism
Fast-Track Strategies For Navigating Abuse

"Only a life lived for others is a life worthwhile."

— Albert Einstein

People who give without expectation live longer, happier lives and make more money. So if we've got a shot at that during our time together, darn it, I'm gonna try.

To make that happen, I have a question for you...

Would you help someone you've never met, even if you never got credit for it?

Who is this person you ask? They are like you. Or, at least, like you used to be. Less experienced, wanting to make a difference, and needing help, but not sure where to look.

My mission is to make Unmask Narcissism accessible to everyone. Everything I do stems from that mission. And, the only way for me to accomplish that mission is by reaching...well...everyone.

This is where you come in. Most people do, in fact, judge a book by its cover (and its reviews). So here's my ask on behalf of a struggling victim of narcissism you've never met:

Please help that struggling victim by leaving this book a review.

To get that 'feel good' feeling and help this person for real, all you have to do is...and it takes less than 60 seconds...

leave a review.

If you feel good about helping a faceless struggling victim, you are my kind of person. Welcome to the club. You're one of us. You'll love the strategies I'm about to share in the coming chapters.

Scan Me

Thank you from the bottom of my heart.
Now, back to our regularly scheduled programming.

- Your biggest fan, Susan Beaumont

PS - Fun fact: If you provide something of value to another person, it makes you more valuable to them. If you'd like goodwill straight from another victim of relationship abuse - and you believe this book will help them - send this book their way!

Chapter 5
Advanced Strategies for High-Conflict Situations

Navigating high-conflict situations with someone who has narcissistic traits can often feel like trying to diffuse a bomb without knowing which wires to cut. The stakes are high, the pressure is on, and the wrong move can escalate things quickly. Understanding the nature of high-conflict personalities, especially those with narcissistic inclinations, is crucial. These individuals thrive on conflict; they see the world as winners and losers and strive to emerge victorious from every interaction. Their behaviors can quickly escalate disputes because their primary concern isn't resolution—it's domination.

5.1 Recognizing the Dynamics: Understanding High-Conflict Personalities

In dealing with such personalities, traditional conflict-resolution tactics, like compromise or mutual understanding, often need to be revised. Instead, advanced de-escalation techniques become your best tools. One effective method is redirecting the conversation away from contentious topics when you sense the tension rising. It's about recognizing when the discussion is veering into dangerous territory and steering it towards safer ground, like a captain navigating stormy seas. For instance, if a conversation with a narcissistic colleague starts to get heated over a project decision, you could shift focus to a related but less controversial topic, like timelines or logistical details, which might diffuse the immediate tension.

5.2 Strategic Engagement: Choosing Your Battles Wisely

Another crucial strategy is choosing your battles wisely. This doesn't mean letting important issues slide but picking moments to engage when and where you can have the most constructive impact. It's about assessing which conflicts are worth your energy and whether a high-conflict personality sets distractions or traps to bait you into a no-win situation. Sometimes, the most potent move in your arsenal is a strategic retreat, preserving your energy for matters where you can effect change.

5.3 Professional and Legal Resources: Seeking Help When Needed

Legal and professional resources become vital when boundary violations escalate into abuse or harassment. Knowing when and how to seek professional help, be it consulting with HR or seeking legal counsel, can provide a safety net when situations deteriorate beyond what can be managed through personal communication alone. For instance, if a narcissistic partner or colleague's actions start impacting your mental health or professional standing, it might be time to take formal steps. Documenting incidents meticulously provides a foundation for your case should you need to take legal action or formally report harassment.

5.4 Self-Preservation: Emotional and Physical Tactics

Self-preservation in high-conflict scenarios involves a combination of emotional and physical tactics. Emotionally, it's crucial to safeguard your inner peace by setting firm mental boundaries and sticking to them.

Dealing with narcissistic behavior can be an exhausting and spiritually draining experience. In these moments, it is essential to remember the power of inner peace. As Philippians 4:7 reminds us,

> *And the peace of God, which transcends all understanding, will guard your hearts and your minds in Christ Jesus.*

By embracing this peace, we can protect ourselves from the chaos that narcissism often brings. When faced with manipulative tactics, take a moment to breathe, pray, and realign with your spiritual center. This inner peace is not a sign of weakness but a profound strength that shields you from the storm.

Techniques such as meditation or therapy can help maintain your equilibrium. Physically, ensuring your safety might mean changing your environment or limiting personal interactions with the high-conflict individual. Deciding to disengage or cut ties, especially in personal relationships, is a complex but sometimes necessary choice for preserving your well-being. It's like realizing that the cost of staying in a toxic dynamic outweighs the potential benefits of resolution.

5.5 Navigating High-Conflict Situations: A Comprehensive Approach

Navigating high-conflict situations with narcissistic personalities requires a blend of courage, strategy, and self-care. You can manage these challenging interactions more effectively by understanding the underlying dynamics, employing targeted de-escalation techniques, utilizing available resources, and prioritizing your safety and well-being. Remember, the goal isn't just to survive; you must also navigate these encounters to preserve your integrity and peace.

In this chapter, we've explored the turbulent waters of dealing with high-conflict personalities, particularly those with narcissistic traits, and provided strategies for maintaining your course through potential storms. From understanding the nature of these conflicts to employing advanced de-escalation tactics and knowing when to seek external support, these tools equip you with the knowledge and skills to handle these dynamics effectively. As we move forward, the focus will shift from managing external conflicts to fostering internal resilience, ensuring that you're not only equipped to handle challenges from others but also empowered to strengthen your own emotional and psychological fortitude.

Chapter 6
Recovery

Imagine you're standing in front of a mirror, not just any mirror, but one that has, for years, reflected a version of you distorted by someone else's narrative. Now, envision replacing that old mirror with one that reflects the actual, unapologetic, and thriving you. This chapter, my dear reader, is about changing out those mirrors. It's about reconstructing the image you see, not through someone else's eyes, but through your own, renewed and clear. This journey of self-love and recovery isn't about getting back to who you were before the narcissistic abuse; it's about discovering who you are now, in the aftermath, and loving that person wholeheartedly.

6.1 Rebuilding Self-Esteem: Exercises and Affirmations

Identifying Negative Self-Talk

First off, let's tackle the pesky critter of negative self-talk. It's like having a mean little gremlin on your shoulder, whispering sweet nothings of the worst kind into your ear. This gremlin grew more loquacious and convincing during your time with a narcissist, echoing their criticisms until you started believing them as gospel truth. But guess what? It's time to silence that gremlin.

Start by catching these negative whispers in the act. Carry a small notebook around, use an app on your phone, and jot down every negative thought about yourself that pops into your head throughout the day. You might write down things like, "I'm not good enough," or "I always mess up." Seeing these thoughts in black and white can be a revelation—it externalizes them and clarifies how harsh you've been on yourself.

Creating Positive Affirmations

Now, for every piece of negative self-talk, let's craft a counteracting affirmation. Affirmations are like your personal cheer squad, rooting for you loudly enough to drown out that gremlin. If you've noted, "I'm not good enough," flip it to, "I am enough, exactly as I am." These affirmations might initially feel awkward or cheesy—like wearing an oversized sweater you need to grow into. But with repetition, they start to fit just right. Repeat them every morning or anytime that gremlin gets chatty. Stick notes on your fridge, mirror, or anywhere you frequently look. Make these positive declarations a part of your daily routine until they become as natural as breathing.

Self-Esteem Boosting Activities

Activities that boost self-esteem are like personal training sessions for your self-worth. Let's get you started on some exercises. Begin with setting small, achievable goals. It could be as simple as cooking a new recipe, finishing a book, or walking daily. Each completed task lets you prove to yourself, "Hey, I can do this!" Also, dive back into old hobbies or explore new ones. Engaging in activities that you enjoy and are good at can significantly bolster your feelings of competence and achievement. Remember, every small win is a brick in the foundation of your rebuilt self-esteem.

Visualization Techniques

Lastly, embrace the power of visualization. This technique is like a rehearsal for your mind, prepping you for upcoming successes. Spend a few minutes each day closing your eyes and vividly imagining achieving your goals. Picture yourself receiving accolades at work, enjoying a hobby, or simply being happy and content. Visualization boosts your mood and reinforces your belief in achieving these realities. It's like sketching out the blueprints for your future successes, making them easier to build when the time comes.

Through these exercises and affirmations, you're not just repairing the old cracks but fortifying your structure, preparing yourself to withstand future storms and dance in the rain. Remember, self-esteem is not static; it's a muscle that needs constant flexing. So, keep at these practices, and watch as the reflection in your new mirror smiles back more brightly each day.

6.2 Rediscovering Joy: Engaging in Self-Love Practices

Think back to when laughter bubbled up effortlessly, where everything seemed to spark a light within you. Maybe it was when you were dabbling in paint, even though the result looked nothing like the picture in your head, or perhaps when you were dancing in your living room, not caring about rhythm or steps. These moments, these joy-filled activities, might feel like echoes of a distant past, especially after the shadow of narcissistic abuse. But what if I told you it's possible to reclaim that joy, to weave it back into the fabric of your daily life? Let's embark on this heartwarming endeavor together, rediscovering what makes your heart sing and sprinkle your days with self-love practices that reignite your inner spark.

First, let's dig up those buried treasures of activities that once brought you joy or might hold the potential to do so. This excavation can be surprisingly delightful. Start by listing things you loved doing as a child or any hobbies you've left behind. Did you enjoy sketching? Singing? Maybe you were captivated by building intricate models or lost in the world of books. Now, think about why you stopped. Time? The narcissist's disdain or mockery? Understanding these blocks can be the first step towards removing them. Next, explore new activities you've never tried but have always been curious about. Pottery? Salsa dancing? Coding? The list is endless, and so are your possibilities. The key is to approach this exploration with the mindset of a curious adventurer. No pressure, just play.

Incorporating these joy practices into your daily routine can transform mundane days into ones sprinkled with anticipation and excitement. It doesn't have to be time-consuming; dedicating a few minutes each day to a beloved hobby or a new interest can significantly boost your mood and overall well-being. Create a joy calendar to schedule daily small activities you look forward to. Monday could be 'meditative coloring day,' Tuesday for 'tending to your garden,' and so on. These activities act like punctuations of joy in your regular schedule, gently reminding you that life is not just about surviving; it's about thriving.

Now, let's talk about the importance of play. Yes, play, like the unstructured, free-form play you indulged in as a kid. It's not frivolous; play is a severe creativity booster and a stress reducer. The play has profound psychological benefits for adults, helping break the shackles of routine and ignite creative thinking. Incorporate play into your life by engaging in activities without rules or objectives—like building a sandcastle, doodling, or dancing freely to your favorite tunes. Play allows you to step outside the structured demands of life, providing a much-needed escape and a powerful tool for stress relief.

Lastly, celebrating yourself should be a regular part of your routine, not just a rare occurrence. Each small achievement on this path of recovery deserves recognition. Have you cooked a meal from scratch? Celebrate it. Have you stood up for yourself in a small way? Pat yourself on the back. These celebrations can be simple, like treating yourself to a nice bath, buying that book you've been eyeing, or just taking a moment to acknowledge your progress. Each celebration is a reaffirmation of your worth and a step towards healing. By recognizing and celebrating each step, no matter how small, you reinforce your achievements and bolster your journey toward a joy-filled, self-loving life.

Engaging in these self-love practices isn't just about filling your days with activities; it's about changing your relationship with yourself. It's about recognizing that you deserve joy, are capable of creativity, and are worthy of celebration. Each step you take in rediscovering joy and engaging in playful activities is a step towards recovering from the past and actively building a vibrant, fulfilling future. Remember, the goal here isn't to return to who you were before the abuse but to evolve into who God made you be—joyful, resilient, and deeply in love with the purposes of your life.

6.3 The Role of Mindfulness in Healing from Abuse

Mindfulness might sound like one of those buzzwords tossed around like confetti these days, but stick with me here. In the context of healing from narcissistic abuse, it's not just a trendy concept; it's a lifeline. At its core, mindfulness is about being fully present in the moment, aware of where we are and what we're doing, without being overly reactive or overwhelmed by what's happening around us. Think of it as learning to sit in the eye of the storm while the winds of past traumas howl around you and, somehow, find a calm space to breathe and be.

For anyone who's felt the chaos of emotional abuse, mindfulness offers a way to regain control over your thoughts and emotions, which have likely been in a perpetual spin cycle. It's about observing these thoughts and feelings without judgment—acknowledging them but not letting them dictate your peace. Imagine you're watching leaves float down a river, each leaf an emotion or a memory. You notice and let them drift by, but you don't jump in the river, and the current pulls you away. This practice can be a powerful tool for grounding yourself in the present, especially when past traumas threaten to pull you back into old, painful patterns.

Mindfulness Exercises

Let's get into some simple exercises designed to anchor you in the here and now, helping to dissipate anxieties and flashbacks triggered by past abuse. A straightforward one is focused breathing. Sit or lie comfortably, close your eyes, and take a deep breath, counting to four. Hold it for a count of four, then exhale for four. Repeat this cycle for a few minutes. It's simple, but you'll be amazed at how it centers your mind and body, pulling your focus back from anxiety-inducing thoughts to the simplicity of your breath.

Another exercise is the sensory check-in, which you can do anywhere, anytime. Pause for a moment, take a few deep breaths, and notice five things you can see, four you can touch, three you can hear, two you can smell, and one you can taste. This exercise helps grounding and sharpen your sensory awareness, rooting you firmly in the present.

Integrating Mindfulness into Daily Life

Incorporating mindfulness into your daily routine can transform it from a practice to a way of life. Start with routine activities like brushing your teeth or washing dishes. Instead of letting your mind wander to yesterday's issues or tomorrow's worries, focus on the sensations and movements involved in the task. Feel the brush in your hand; notice the foam and strokes. It's a practice of keeping your mind from straying into troubled waters and training it to stay anchored in the present.

You can also use mindfulness during more emotionally charged moments, which are especially common as you navigate the road to recovery from abuse. When you feel old triggers surfacing, take a mindful moment to pause and breathe, acknowledge the emotions without judgment, and gently guide your focus back to your current activity. This practice can help prevent the spiraling of emotions, allowing you to respond to situations rather than react impulsively.

Help prevent the spiraling of emotions, allowing you to respond to situations rather than react impulsively.

Mindfulness and Emotional Regulation

One of the greatest gifts of mindfulness in the context of recovering from abuse is its ability to help regulate emotions. For someone healing from narcissistic abuse, emotional regulation can often feel like trying to lasso a tornado. Mindfulness steadies this whirlwind, not by suppressing emotions but by allowing them space to be acknowledged and understood. This understanding fosters a better management of emotional responses.

For instance, when a wave of anger or sadness washes over you, instead of immediately reacting or pushing it away, mindfulness teaches you to recognize the emotion, explore its origins, and let it pass without letting it overwhelm you. It's about acknowledging that while you may not have control over everything that happens to you, you do have control over how you respond. Over time, this leads to a more balanced emotional life, turning what once felt like an emotional battlefield into a more navigable landscape.

As you integrate these mindfulness practices into your life, they become less of exercises and more of a way of being. This shift doesn't just help you cope with the aftermath of narcissistic abuse; it empowers you to lead a life defined not by what you've endured but by the peace and presence you cultivate every day. As you continue to practice mindfulness, remember that each moment of awareness is a step away from the past and a step towards a centered, peaceful, and present you.

6.4 Creating a Self-Care Routine: A Step-by-Step Guide

Let's talk about self-care. Not the trendy kind, with its face masks and bubble baths (though don't get me wrong, those are fantastic!), but the type of deep, nourishing self-care that rebuilds your sense of self and personal agency after experiencing narcissistic abuse. Think of it as constructing your sanctuary, where you are safe, valued, and cared for—by you, for you. Self-care in this context is about more than just feeling good; it's about cultivating practices that restore and maintain your mental, physical, and emotional health, providing a foundation for the vibrant life you deserve.

The Importance of Self-Care in Recovery

Imagine your energy as a personal currency. In a relationship with a narcissist, you likely spend this currency in vast amounts, often receiving little to nothing in return. Now, as you recover, think of self-care as the most profitable investment you can make in your bank of well-being. It's about paying yourself first and ensuring you replenish and enrich your energy reserves. Practicing self-care helps you regain control over your health and emotions, reconstructing your sense of self that was eroded by the narcissist's influence. It's like telling yourself, "I matter. My well-being matters," and proving it through actions.

Components of a Self-Care Routine

A robust self-care routine encompasses physical, mental, and emotional practices. Physically, it could be as simple as integrating regular movement into your day. This doesn't necessarily mean running marathons (unless that's your thing!), but finding physical activities that you enjoy and that nourish your body—yoga, dancing in your living room, or just stretching in the morning sun. Mentally, self-care might involve engaging in activities that stimulate your mind and distract you from ruminative thoughts. Puzzle games, reading, or learning a new skill can all be part of this. Emotionally, self-care practices might include setting aside time for reflective journaling, seeking therapeutic help, or simply ensuring you have regular, hearty laughs.

Tailoring Self-Care to Individual Needs

No one-size-fits-all approach exists for effective self-care because no one-size-fits-all person exists. Your self-care routine should be as unique as you are, tailored to fit your needs and your preferences, lifestyle, and circumstances. Start by assessing your current state: How are you feeling physically? Drained? Restless? What about emotionally? Anxious? Numb? Your answers will guide you in choosing practices that address your immediate needs. For instance, if you're feeling isolated, your self-care might focus on reconnecting with old friends or joining new groups that share your interests. If you're physically exhausted, it might be time to consider your sleep hygiene or nutritional choices.

Commitment to Self-Care

Committing to a self-care routine is like making a promise to your future self to keep putting your well-being on the top of your priority list. Start small; overwhelming yourself with an elaborate routine might lead to frustration. Set reminders on your phone for time-outs, just brief moments initially, where you engage in your chosen self-care activity. Involve supportive friends or family by sharing your self-care goals with them; they can offer encouragement and hold you accountable. Tracking your progress can also be incredibly motivating. Whether marking a calendar for every day you meet your self-care goals or keeping a journal detailing how you feel before and after your self-care practices, seeing your progress can reinforce the value of these activities, encouraging you to stick with them.

In weaving these self-care threads into the fabric of your daily life, you're not just healing from past abuse; you're building a new, healthier framework for your life. Each act of self-care is a step towards regaining your autonomy and reinforcing the truth that you are worthy of care and love—most notably, from yourself.

6.5 Embracing Solitude for Emotional Recovery

Let's chat about solitude. Often, solitude gets a bad rap, painted in shades of loneliness and as a sign of social unpopularity. But what if we flipped the script? Imagine solitude not as a barren island but as a personal sanctuary, a space where you can meet your true self away from the noise and demands of the world. This reimagining is crucial, especially after experiencing the turbulence of a relationship marred by narcissism, where the needs and manipulations of another might have constantly overshadowed your thoughts and feelings.

Solitude offers a rare, undiluted form of freedom. It provides the quiet needed to sift through your thoughts, understand your feelings, and truly make your own decisions. Think of it as having a coffee date with yourself, where the conversation can meander through topics without interruption, judgment, or influence. This can be incredibly healing. It's in these moments of self-reflection that you can begin to untangle the threads of your narrative from the suffocating weave of the narcissistic relationship.

Now, what does productive solitude look like? It's anything that nurtures your spirit and refocuses your energy inward. Journaling is a fantastic tool. It allows you to dialogue with yourself, posing questions and exploring answers that might surprise you. Each page can serve as a stepping stone away from past pain. Consider setting aside a few minutes each day to write freely. Don't worry about grammar or coherence—let your thoughts flow as they will. This practice isn't just about reflection; it's a process of reclaiming your voice.

Meditative walks are another enriching solitary activity. Walking alone provides a rhythmic backdrop for introspection, Whether a stroll through a park or along a city sidewalk. With each step, imagine walking away from past hurts, and towards a future you define. Use this time to connect with nature, to feel the sun or the breeze, to hear the crunch of leaves underfoot, or to hear the distant murmur of city life. These sensory experiences can ground you in the present, helping to clear the mental clutter left by years of manipulation.

Creative arts offer a third avenue for productive solitude. Creative activities can be meditative, whether you're painting, playing an instrument, or knitting. They focus your mind and keep your hands busy, physically manifesting your inner state. There's something profoundly therapeutic about watching a piece of art take shape under your hands, a tangible reminder that you can create beauty from within, regardless of external circumstances.

Building comfort with being alone doesn't happen overnight, especially if your past relationship has made you equate being alone with being unloved or unwanted. Start small. Spend a few minutes alone without distractions—no phone, TV, just you. Gradually increase this time as your comfort level grows. This practice helps to deconstruct your negative associations with being alone, teaching you that solitude can be a peaceful, not painful, experience.

Solitude, when embraced, can be a powerful tool in your recovery arsenal. It allows deep self-reflection free from outside influence, providing the quiet to listen to and understand your deepest thoughts and feelings. In these quiet moments, you can start to process and heal from the emotional turmoil caused by narcissistic abuse. You learn that being alone doesn't mean being lonely; it means being with yourself, fully and completely, perhaps for the first time in a long time. This reconnection with your inner self is a critical step in healing that reaffirms your worth and independence outside any relationship.

In this sacred space of solitude, you're not just spending time alone but investing in a deeper understanding and appreciation of yourself. You're learning that your own company is not just enough; it's enriching. This transformation in how you view and value your alone time is not just about recovery; it's about empowerment. It's a vital part of rediscovering and reaffirming who you are, what you need, and what you no longer will accept. Embrace solitude not as a sign of isolation but as a celebration of self-discovery and self-respect.

6.6 Celebrating Small Wins: Tracking Progress on Your Journey

Let's think about recovery as a garden you're tending. Every bit of effort, no matter how minor it seems, contributes to the overall beauty of your garden. Small wins in your recovery are like those little seeds you plant; each one has the potential to grow into something magnificent. But first, let's define what a 'small win' could look like for someone coming out of the fog of narcissistic abuse. It might be as simple as setting a boundary and sticking to it, or it could be a day when the shadow of guilt didn't darken your doorstep. Perhaps it was saying no to an unreasonable request, or maybe it was just getting out of bed when depression wanted you to stay tucked under the covers.

Recognizing and celebrating these wins is crucial, not because they're steps toward returning to 'normal'—whatever that may mean—but because they affirm your growth and resilience. Now, how do we keep track of these wins? One delightful way is through journaling. Think of your journal as a garden log where you note what seeds you've planted and how they're doing. Whenever you jot down a small win, you're documenting your growth. This can be incredibly validating when it feels like you haven't made progress, reminding you of how far you've come.

Another vibrant method is creating a 'victory wall'—a physical or digital space where you post notes, photos, or artifacts of your achievements. This could be sticky notes on your bedroom wall or a dedicated folder on your computer. Each item on this wall represents a win; collectively, they tell the story of your healing journey.

It's a visual celebration of your resilience, a daily reminder that you are progressing despite the challenges.

The psychological impact of acknowledging these small wins is profound. Each acknowledgment acts like sunlight in your garden, nurturing your self-esteem and motivation. It's based on positive reinforcement—the more you recognize your efforts, the more motivated you'll feel to continue. This is crucial during recovery, as it helps shift your focus from what's been lost to what's being gained. It transforms recovery from a daunting task into a rewarding process, where each small win adds a layer of strength to your newfound resilience.

Sharing these successes with trusted friends or support groups can amplify their power. When others celebrate with you, they acknowledge your progress, validate your experience, and reinforce your sense of accomplishment. This external validation can be incredibly supportive, especially when self-doubt creeps in. It serves as a reminder that others see, value, and support your efforts, further strengthening your commitment to your recovery path.

In nurturing your recovery garden, remember that every small win deserves recognition. Whether it's a sprout of new growth or a fully blooming flower, each is a testament to your resilience and commitment to reclaiming your life. As you continue to tend this garden, let each small win remind you of your strength and your capacity to thrive, not just despite your past experiences but because of how you've chosen to grow from them.

As we wrap up this chapter on self-love and recovery, remember that this process is less about reaching a destination and more about appreciating the journey—each step, each win, each moment of joy. You are not just recovering; you are rediscovering and redefining who you are. This chapter celebrates that process, recognizing the strength it takes to rebuild and the beauty of nurturing your well-being. As we move forward, carry with you the lessons of self-care, the practices of mindfulness, and the joy of small victories. Let them guide you as you cultivate a life of resilience, happiness, and profound self-love.

Chapter 7
Practical Advice for Exiting Toxic Relationships

Picture this: you're standing at the edge of an emotional cliff. Behind you lies a turbulent sea of toxic dynamics, and the solid ground of a healthier life beckons ahead. It's not just a step; it's a leap towards your freedom, your peace, and a bit of the unknown. Deciding to leave a toxic relationship is no small feat. It's a testament to your strength, even if your knees feel wobbly at the thought. But like any significant life change, the devil is in the details. This chapter is your map through the minefield, equipped with humor, empathy, and practical steps to ensure your journey toward safety and readiness isn't just a leap of faith but a jump of informed strategic action.

7.1 Preparing to Leave: A Checklist for Safety and Readiness

Safety Planning

Let's talk safety first because it's the bedrock of your leap. Think of it as packing your parachute carefully before the jump. Crafting a detailed safety plan is paramount, especially in the unpredictable landscape of a toxic relationship. This plan is your private blueprint, so confidentiality is critical. Start by gathering all essential documents—birth certificates, passports, social security cards. Have them ready in a 'go bag,' maybe tucked away with a trusted friend or in a secure, quickly accessible place.

Next, secure alternative accommodation. Whether it's a friend's couch, a family member's spare room, or a shelter, ensure you have a safe landing spot for the initial days or weeks post-departure. And here's where your support network comes into play. Inform them of your plans where safe to do so; their support can be a lifeline in times of uncertainty. If possible, establish coded language or signals to communicate distress or the need to enact your exit plan without alerting the narcissist.

Emotional Readiness

Now, steeling your nerves is easier said than done, right? Emotional readiness is like rehearsing your lines before opening night. Feeling a whirlwind of emotions, from fear to guilt to relief, is expected. Lean into these feelings with the support of counseling or therapy. Professionals help fortify your emotional armor, ensuring you're psychologically prepared for the challenges during and after your departure.

Keep your focus laser-sharp on the reasons you're leaving. Write them down, talk them over with a therapist, chant them as a mantra—whatever keeps the flame of resolve lit. The narcissist will try to blow out that flame with emotional manipulation. Your preparedness is the glass shield protecting your resolve from their gusts.

Timing Considerations

Timing is not just about finding the right moment; it's about strategic planning. Aim for a time when the narcissist is least likely to be around, reducing the immediate risk of confrontation. It could be during their regular gym time or a weekend retreat they always attend. The less dramatic the exit, the safer you'll be. Also, consider the logistical aspects of moving out. If you can, arrange for help from friends or a moving service at a time when interference is least likely.

Confidentiality and Digital Security

In the digital age, a digital footprint can be a breadcrumb trail back to you, so tightening up digital security is crucial. Change passwords on your personal accounts—email, social media, banking—and, if possible, do so from a device the narcissist doesn't have access to. Consider a new, secure email account for the most sensitive communications about your plans. Also, review your social media privacy settings or take a hiatus from platforms to avoid inadvertently providing clues about your whereabouts or plans.

Navigating the departure from a toxic relationship is undeniably complex and fraught with emotional and practical challenges. But with careful planning, emotional preparation, and strategic timing, you can ensure that your exit is not just a flight toward safety but a gateway to a new chapter of freedom and healing. Remember, each step, each plan, and each discreet preparation is a stitch in the fabric of your new life, woven with threads of courage, hope, and the support of those who believe in your right to a healthier, happier existence.

7.2 Legal Considerations: Protecting Yourself and Your Assets

Stepping away from a toxic relationship isn't just an emotional rollercoaster—it's a legal labyrinth, too, especially when tangled assets and, heaven forbid, custody issues enter the mix. Think of this as untangling two lives and ensuring you walk away with your legal rights intact and your future secured. Let's slice through the legal jargon and make this as painless as possible.

First things first, cozy up with a lawyer who gets it. I mean, someone who understands the ins and outs of domestic issues, not just someone who can spell 'divorce.' A good lawyer isn't just a legal defender; they're your strategic ally in what can often feel like a chess game where the stakes are your future. They can guide you through the necessary steps to protect yourself, from filing for restraining orders if your safety is threatened to navigating the murky waters of legal battles that might arise. It's like having a legal GPS during a particularly nasty storm.

Now, onto documenting abuse. If the walls of your home could talk, what tales would they tell? Since they can't, this burden rests on your shoulders. Documenting instances of abuse isn't just cathartic—it's critical. Keep a detailed log of dates, times, incidents, and witnesses. Store any threatening texts, emails, or voicemails. This evidence can be crucial in court, clearly showing what you've endured. Think of it as gathering ammo for a battle you never wanted to fight. Keep these records in a safe place—perhaps with a trusted friend or in a locked file—if you worry about them being discovered.

Understanding marital assets can feel like you're trying to split the sea. Whether it's who gets the house or how to handle joint accounts, the details matter. Before you make any moves, get clear on what's shared and what's yours. It's not just about fairness; it's about ensuring you don't walk away empty-handed from years spent building a life together. Legal advice is priceless here. A financial affidavit might become your new best friend, detailing everything from your coffee spoons to your savings accounts. Your lawyer can help you navigate this, ensuring you get your equitable share without overstepping legal boundaries.

If little ones are in the picture, the plot, as they say, thickens. Child custody considerations are about putting their well-being front and center. It's a delicate dance of legal rights and emotional needs. Your lawyer can help craft a custody arrangement that shields your kids from the toxic behaviors of a narcissistic parent. This might involve supervised visits or detailed parenting plans that specify pickup and drop-off routines, communication guidelines, and even rules around new partners. It's about creating a buffer zone where your children can thrive, even when navigating the divided loyalties of separated parents.

Navigating these legal waters requires a cool head and a clear strategy supported by professional advice and meticulous preparation. Whether securing your assets or protecting your children, the legal system offers tools and protections designed to help you turn the page on this chapter safely and securely. With the proper preparation and support, you can step into this legal arena confident, prepared, and ready to start anew, knowing that you've done everything within your power to pave the way for a brighter, safer future.

7.3 Financial Independence: Strategies for Economic Empowerment

Imagine you're embarking on a road trip to a place you've always wanted to explore. The journey is thrilling, but you must have enough fuel, a reliable map, and perhaps some good tunes. Similarly, stepping out of a narcissistic relationship into a life of independence is an exhilarating journey that requires financial planning, resources, and, yes, a bit of that 'can-do' soundtrack to keep you motivated. Let's dig into how you can secure your financial independence, ensuring you have the means to support your new circumstances, protect your assets, and confidently navigate the road ahead.

Assessing Financial Status

First things first, let's assess where you stand financially. It's like taking a snapshot of your current financial health. How much do you have in your bank accounts? Are there debts nipping at your heels? What about assets—things you own that add value to your financial pot, like a car or jewelry? And let's not forget about potential resources you might tap into, perhaps a savings bond you forgot about or a family member who's been nudging you to accept some help.

Creating a budget is your next step, and it's more manageable than it sounds. Simply list your income sources, then tally up your expenses—everything from your morning coffee to your mortgage. This visual representation will clarify where your money is going and where you might tighten up, ensuring your financial ship doesn't spring any leaks. Remember, a budget isn't set in stone; it's a living document that adjusts as your life changes. It's your financial heartbeat; keep a close watch on it.

Building Financial Reserves

Now, let's talk about building your financial reserves—think of it as your safety net, designed to catch you if you stumble during your leap to independence. Opening a separate bank account is a stealthy first step. It's not just about secrecy; it's about having a financial space under your control, with no strings attached. Start funneling a portion of your income into this account. Even small amounts can snowball into a substantial buffer over time, giving you the financial stamina to withstand and recover from setbacks without relying on your former partner.

Understanding the financial implications of separation or divorce is crucial. If you're married, this might mean untangling joint accounts or deciding who gets the espresso machine. It's about ensuring you walk away with your fair share, equipped to start afresh. Fair share might involve negotiations or legal consultations, but every step you take builds a sturdier financial foundation for your new life.

Credit Protection

Protecting and rebuilding your credit score during and after leaving a narcissistic relationship is like polishing your armor—it's protective and empowering. Start by pulling your credit report.

Check for any joint accounts or loans that might impact your credit. If your narcissistic partner was less than responsible with shared credit, you might find some unpleasant surprises. Address this head-on by contacting creditors to close or separate joint accounts or refinancing loans only in your name.

Building your credit independently involves making timely payments, even on the most minor bills, and keeping your credit utilization low. Consider a secured credit card if you need to build your credit from scratch. It's like training wheels for your credit score, helping you gain momentum safely.

Seeking Financial Advice

Lastly, don't go it alone. Consulting with financial advisors or support services can provide personalized guidance tailored to your unique situation. These experts can offer strategies and insights that turn complex financial jargon into actionable steps. Whether it's navigating the intricacies of a financial separation or planning for long-term financial goals, their advice can be a lighthouse guiding you through murky waters.

Embracing financial independence when stepping out of a narcissistic relationship is about more than just dollars and cents—it's about reclaiming your autonomy and ensuring your financial decisions support your life's goals and dreams. With careful planning, a clear understanding of your financial landscape, and the proper support, you can turn financial independence from a daunting challenge into an empowering achievement, laying a solid foundation for your journey toward a secure and fulfilling future.

7.4 Finding and Using Support Systems Effectively

Imagine you're at a crossroads, with the path behind you tangled with the thorns of a toxic relationship and the roads ahead leading to potential new beginnings. At this juncture, having a network of supporters—friends who arm you with comfort, family who shield you with love, or community resources that light your path—can make all the difference. Let's unfold the map of support systems, identifying who and what can be your allies in this transformative phase of your life.

Firstly, let's talk about friends and family. They're like your personal cheer squad, right? But here's the catch: not all teams can handle the playoffs. It's vital to identify which members of your circle genuinely understand the dynamics of abusive relationships and are capable of offering the support you need. This chosen group isn't just about who can offer a shoulder to cry on; it's about who can keep confidence, provide wise counsel without judgment, and stand by you steadfastly as you navigate your exit. Think of each person's strengths and limitations. Aunt Joan might be great for a night out to distract you, but she might not be the best at keeping secrets. Your friend from yoga, however, might be a great confidant who keeps grounded in stressful times.

Moving beyond your immediate circle, consider the power of community resources. Shelters, legal aid, and financial counseling services are like the hidden tracks on a favorite album—there when you need them, offering specialized help tailored to situations like yours. These resources often provide anonymity and safety, crucial elements when you're planning an escape from a narcissist's influence. Engaging with these services can offer a structured, professional support system that complements the emotional support of friends and family. For instance, shelters not only provide a temporary safe space but can also connect you to legal advice and therapeutic services to start healing from abuse.

Professional support from therapists or counselors specializing in dealing with trauma and abusive relationships is like having a guide in a foreign city. They can help navigate the complex emotions and situations when leaving a toxic relationship. These professionals can offer strategies for emotional distancing, advice on legal protections, and therapeutic techniques to rebuild your sense of self-worth and autonomy. Their external, unbiased perspective can be invaluable, especially when your perspective may be clouded by manipulation and gaslighting.

Maintaining privacy while engaging with these support systems is crucial, especially when the risk of interference from a narcissist looms large. It's like setting up a firewall; you protect your plans and emotional space from hacking. When reaching out for support, whether online or in person, use secure methods of communication. Consider setting up new email accounts or social media profiles, and always be cautious about sharing details related to you. If attending support groups or therapy, ensure these meetings are in secure, confidential locations where you won't be observed or followed. This level of caution helps maintain the integrity of your support network, keeping it a safe and effective tool in your recovery and escape.

As you map out your support network, remember that each person and resource adds a layer of strength to your foundation. They collectively create a web of safety and affirmation, crucial for anyone stepping away from the shadows of abuse into the light of self-reclaimed life. Engage with these supports actively, maintain your privacy fiercely, and use their strengths wisely to bolster your journey to independence and peace.

7.5 Coping with Loneliness Post-Separation

When you've finally turned the page on a relationship that's been more draining than a marathon episode of a tear-jerker series, the silence in its aftermath can be deafening. It's you, your thoughts, and maybe a few echoes of what used to be. While a relief in some senses, this solitude can usher in a visitor named Loneliness that you didn't invite. It's normal to feel this void where drama once lived. It's like finishing a long, intense book series—what do you do now? First, breathe. Loneliness is not a sign of doing something wrong; it's a natural part of recalibrating your emotional life.

Let's sprinkle a little fun into this mix. Engaging in new activities can be your way of rewriting your day-to-day script. Have you ever thought about line dancing? What about painting or joining a bowling league? These aren't just fillers but bridges to new interests and connections. Each step into something new is a step away from the old, the one that didn't cheer for you. Activities that pique your interest are more than distractions—they're pathways to healing. They connect you with like-minded souls, maybe even those who've walked paths similar to yours, who understand that sometimes you just need to say, "Hey, this sucks," and have someone nod back with genuine understanding.

Therapy, too, can be an incredible resource during this time. It's not just about talking—it's about unpacking. Sometimes, you don't even know the weight you've been carrying until you start laying it out on the table, piece by piece, in front of someone trained to help you sort through it. Therapists can guide you through the loneliness, help you understand it, and give you tools to build a new, healthier emotional life. They're like the GPS when you find yourself in the wilds of your emotions—turn left here, keep going straight, and watch out for that old thinking pattern ahead. And support groups? They're like group road trips on this journey. Sharing with others, who nod and understand because they've seen that same rocky landscape, can make all the difference.

As for your social life, think of it as a garden. It's time to tend it, maybe replant it. Rebuilding old friendships can be as comforting as a favorite old sweater but also requires a gentle touch. People change, and so have you, especially after navigating a relationship that's been all-consuming. Reach out, reconnect, and share your story, but also listen. Remember, these are relationships, not just touchpoints for your healing. They require give and take. Nurturing new relationships, meanwhile, should be about setting new patterns. Choose people who uplift, understand boundaries, and share your values—people who laugh with you, not at you. These choices are not just about filling up your social calendar; it's about writing a new narrative where you surround yourself with support and positivity.

Embracing this post-separation period as a time of growth can transform loneliness from a shadow into a signpost that points toward new, enriching experiences and relationships. It's about turning the page, not just with hope, but with a plan and actions that affirm your path to a fulfilled and joyful life.

7.6 Managing Communication with a Narcissist Post-Breakup

Navigating communication with a narcissist after you've taken the courageous step to end the relationship can feel like trying to disarm a bomb without setting it off. You're aiming for peace and minimal drama, but you're dealing with someone who might use every interaction to pull you back into the chaos. Here's how to manage this tricky terrain: setting firm boundaries, using mediated communication, documenting everything, and never hesitating to lean on your support system.

When setting strict communication boundaries, think of it as creating a protective bubble around your emotional space. This emotional space is essential when you cannot cut off communication, such as co-parenting. Keep interactions brief, factual, and devoid of any emotional charge. Pretend you're a diplomat: your words are polite but measured, your emotions are checked at the door, and every interaction is purposeful. Define clear limits on the topic of discussion. For instance, if your communication is for co-parenting, keep the conversation strictly about the kids. Discuss pick-up times, health issues, or school events, but avoid personal topics that could lead to conflict.

Mediated communication can be a game-changer, especially in sticky situations where emotions can flare easily. Technology can be your ally here. Consider using communication services or software designed for high-conflict scenarios, particularly those that keep records of all exchanges. Apps designed for co-parenting can be handy as they log messages, cannot be deleted, and are admissible in court if needed. This tool helps keep communication clean and task-oriented and provides a layer of protection should you need evidence of inappropriate or aggressive exchanges.

Documenting interactions might sound over the top, but it's a crucial step in managing post-breakup communications with a narcissist. Think of it as keeping receipts—you hope you never need them, but you'll be glad to have them if you do. Keep logs of all communications, including texts, emails, and even phone calls. Note the date, time, and content. If things ever escalate, these records can be invaluable in legal settings, providing clear evidence of behavior patterns and helping to enforce boundaries legally. More importantly, if your ex ever tries to gaslight you or twist the narrative, you have your unalterable record of events.

Lastly, navigating this post-breakup communication maze is not a solo journey—rely on your support network. This network should include close friends, family members, a therapist, or legal counsel. They can offer emotional support, perspective, and advice if you're unsure how to handle a tricky interaction. Don't underestimate the value of a quick check-in with a friend before you send a message or the peace of mind that comes from discussing a disturbing exchange with your therapist. They can help you stay grounded and focused, reminding you why maintaining these boundaries is essential for your well-being.

Navigating the choppy waters of post-breakup communications with a narcissist requires a clear strategy, a cool head, and a steadfast commitment to protecting your emotional health. By setting strict boundaries, utilizing mediated communication tools, meticulously documenting interactions, and leaning on your support system, you can manage these necessary exchanges without getting pulled back into turmoil. Each careful step in this process is a reaffirmation of your independence and a testament to your resilience.

As this chapter closes, remember that managing communication with a narcissist post-breakup is about maintaining your dignity and safeguarding your emotional well-being. The strategies discussed here are more than just tactics; they are affirmations of your autonomy, tools that empower you to navigate this complex terrain confidently. As we turn the page, the journey continues, building on these foundations to explore further aspects of healing and growth post-narcissistic abuse.

Chapter 8
Healing and Moving Forward

Imagine stepping into a vast library, each book a different narrative on healing and personal growth. Here, in the quiet comfort of these imagined sacred halls, you're about to pick the book that resonates most deeply with your current chapter in life. This part of your story is about healing and moving forward, learning to weave the threads of your experiences into a stronger fabric of self. It's about transforming the painful past into a narrative of empowerment and hope.

8.1 Therapy Options: Finding the Right Help for You

Navigating the world of therapy can sometimes feel like trying to choose a course at a gourmet restaurant without a menu—overwhelming, right? Let's simplify the menu by exploring the various types of therapy available, each offering unique flavors and benefits, especially when recovering from narcissistic abuse.

Understanding Different Therapy Modalities

Cognitive-behavioral therapy (CBT) is like having a personal trainer for your brain, helping you challenge and change unhelpful cognitive distortions and behaviors, improve emotional regulation, and develop personal coping strategies. It's particularly effective if you find yourself stuck in negative thinking patterns resulting from the abuse.

Dialectical behavior therapy (DBT), on the other hand, emphasizes the psychosocial aspects of treatment. Think of DBT as your mindfulness guru, teaching you how to live in the moment, cope healthily with stress, regulate your emotions, and improve relationships with others. It's especially beneficial if emotional swings have become a frequent visitor.

Trauma-focused therapy is akin to a deep-sea diving expedition, exploring the depths of your emotional psyche to confront and heal from the trauma directly. It uses various techniques to help you process and make sense of your past experiences, which is crucial for those who have survived long-term narcissistic abuse.

Choosing the Right Therapist

Selecting a therapist is more intimate than picking out a new doctor. You want someone who isn't just qualified but also someone you feel comfortable with, almost as if you're choosing a partner for a journey through your inner landscape. Look for therapists who specialize in narcissistic abuse and personality disorders, as they can offer tailored strategies that are aware of the nuances of your experiences. A good fit feels like conversing with an old friend with much expertise in helping you heal.

Accessibility of Therapy

Therapy should not be a luxury item. If budget constraints are a concern, look for therapists who offer sliding scale fees based on your income. Many community mental health centers provide services at reduced rates or even for free. Additionally, online therapy platforms can be more affordable and flexible, allowing you to receive help from the comfort of your home.

Reflection Section

Take a moment to reflect on what you most want to gain from therapy. Are the expectations strategies to handle specific symptoms, tools to rebuild your self-esteem, or guidance on establishing healthy relationships? Writing down your goals can help you clarify your needs and maximize therapy.

Expectations from Therapy

Setting realistic expectations is like putting your seatbelt on a roller coaster—it doesn't stop the ups and downs but ensures you stay secure throughout the ride. Therapy is not a magic cure; it's a healing process that requires active participation and can sometimes feel like two steps forward and one step back. It involves time and emotional investment, and progress might feel slow. But remember, even small steps are still moving forward.

Embarking on therapy is a significant step toward reclaiming your life and narrative from the shadows of narcissistic abuse. It provides a structured environment to understand and heal from your experiences, offering tools and insights that foster long-term healing and resilience. As you explore these therapeutic paths, remember that it's not just about finding the proper help—it's also about becoming the hero of your own story, one where you emerge healed and whole.

8.2 Support Groups and Community: Leveraging Collective Wisdom

Imagine you're at a giant potluck dinner, where everyone brings a dish to share. Some dishes are sweet, some are savory, and some are a bit of both. In this analogy, the dishes represent the diverse experiences and insights everyone brings to a support group. These groups are like a feast for the soul, where shared experiences and collective wisdom can nourish your healing process. Whether it's an online forum buzzing with activity or a quiet local meetup, the essence of these gatherings is the realization that you're not alone in your struggles.

Benefits of Support Groups

The power of shared experiences in support groups is mighty. There's something profoundly comforting about being in a room, virtual or otherwise, with people who nod and understand what you mean when you talk about the confusion and pain caused by narcissistic abuse. It's not just about not feeling alone; it's about feeling understood. This understanding fosters a unique emotional support that feels like a warm blanket on a cold night. Furthermore, these groups provide a platform for exchanging coping strategies. What worked for one person might just work for you or inspire a new approach you hadn't considered. And let's not forget the empowerment that comes from helping others through sharing your own stories—even as you help, you heal.

Finding the Right Group

Looking for the right support group can feel like dating—you might need to try a few before you find the custom fit. Start with online searches for local groups or check platforms like Meetup. Online forums can be a great alternative if you're not ready to attend physical meetings. Websites like Reddit and Facebook host myriad support groups where anonymity can make it easier to start talking. Therapist-led groups might be the ticket for those who prefer a more structured environment. These groups often provide peer support and professional guidance, making them a robust space for recovery.

Interactive Element: Group Finder Checklist

To make your search easier, here's a simple checklist:

- **Determine Your Comfort Level:** Decide if you prefer face-to-face interaction or the anonymity of online forums.
- **Ask About Structure:** Some groups are more structured and led by professionals; others are more casual, peer-led discussions.
- **Check Accessibility:** Ensure the meeting times and locations (or online platform accessibility) fit your schedule.
- **Understand Privacy Policies:** Especially online, understand how your data and information will be protected.

Role of Community in Healing

Spiritual strength can be a guiding light when healing. Seek out a church family that aligns with your current understanding of God, one where you can grow spiritually at a pace that feels right for you.

The broader community plays an essential role in your healing journey. Beyond support groups, community resources like workshops, seminars, and local library events can offer educational opportunities and additional support networks. Engaging in community activities can also provide a sense of normalcy and routine, which is crucial when your world feels like it's turned upside down. Whether it's a community-run mental health day, a workshop on self-care techniques, or regular meetups with people sharing similar experiences, every interaction strengthens your recovery web.

Etiquette and Boundaries in Groups

While support groups are invaluable, maintaining privacy and respect is crucial. It's important to remember that everyone is in a different stage of their healing. A small step for one could be a giant leap for another. Always listen as much as you speak, and respect the confidentiality of sharing in the group. Similarly, set boundaries for your sharing. It's okay not to divulge everything; share what feels comfortable. Establishing these boundaries makes support groups a safe space for everyone, ensuring that the shared wisdom does more than just inform—it heals.

In these gatherings, whether they echo with laughter or heavy with shared sorrow, the collective wisdom of support groups and community resources provides a compass to guide you through the fog of recovery. Each story shared, each hand extended in understanding, and each nod of recognition lights your path a little more, reminding you that on this road, you walk together.

8.3 Steps to Forgiveness

Breaking down the forgiveness process can make it more approachable, even manageable. Start by acknowledging the hurt. Sit with it, understand how deeply it's embedded in your emotions, and recognize how it has affected you. Breaking down the forgiveness might feel like reopening old wounds, but it's the first step in healing them. Acknowledgment validates your feelings, affirming that they matter and that what happened was not okay. This step alone can be liberating.

Next, try to understand the impact of the hurt. How has it shaped your view of yourself and others? How has it influenced your behaviors and your relationships? This understanding of the impact isn't about dredging up pain for pain's sake but tracing the roots of your wounds so you can effectively address them. It's akin to understanding why a plant might be wilting—the better you know the cause, the more effectively you can nurture it back to health.

The decision to forgive is the pivotal moment in this process. It's a conscious choice, often made not once but repeatedly, as old pains resurface and challenge your resolve. Forgiving doesn't mean condoning the abuse; you are choosing to reclaim your power. It's a commitment to stop letting past hurts dictate your emotional state and to start healing on your terms. God tells his people (Isaiah 43:18-19) to not remember the past and to embrace what they can change.

Forgiveness and Reconciliation

It's crucial to differentiate between forgiveness and reconciliation. Forgiving someone does not automatically entail re-establishing a relationship. You can forgive someone and choose not to have them in your life. Reconciliation is a separate process that involves two willing parties and a mutual commitment to rebuild trust and resolve past hurts. It should only be considered if it's safe and healthy for you and if the other party has shown genuine remorse and a commitment to change.

In cases of narcissistic abuse, reconciliation might not be safe or possible, as it requires a level of empathy and willingness to change that narcissists often do not possess. Forgiveness is still valuable for personal peace, but it is more about your healing than mending the relationship.

Forgiving someone who has deeply hurt you, primarily through manipulation and deceit, is one of the toughest challenges you might face. But when approached as a process for your benefit, it becomes a powerful act of self-love. It's about giving yourself the permission to move forward, unburdened by past pains, free to cultivate joy, peace, and healthier relationships on your terms. As you navigate this process, be gentle with yourself, allowing the time and space you need to heal, grow, and eventually, let go.

8.4 Lessons Learned: How to Spot Red Flags in Future Relationships

Navigating the landscape of new relationships after experiencing narcissistic abuse is akin to walking through a beautiful garden laced with hidden thorns. You want to enjoy the blooming flowers —the potential of new connections—but you also know the pain of pricking your finger all too well. Let's talk about spotting those thorns early, not to dampen the joy of new relationships but to ensure you can fully enjoy the garden without harm.

Identifying Red Flags

Red flags in relationships are like warning signals blinking on your car's dashboard; they alert you before a minor issue becomes a major problem. In relationships, some red flags are universally recognized: excessive charm can sometimes be a mask that hides deeper insecurities or manipulative tendencies. It's that over-the-top flattery that feels too good to be true, often used by individuals who want to gain your trust and affection quickly.

Rapid commitment is another pulsing red light. Think of it as someone trying to speed up the relationship timeline excessively, declaring love, pushing for exclusivity, or moving in together surprisingly fast. This tactic will deeply entangle you in the relationship before you can see their true colors.

Lastly, a disregard for boundaries is a critical red flag. If someone consistently pushes past your comfort zone, ignoring your expressed wishes and testing the limits you've set, it's a clear sign of disrespect for your autonomy. Whether it's bombarding you with texts when you've asked for space or insisting on discussing topics you've marked as off-limits, these are signs that they do not value your boundaries, which is a cornerstone of any healthy relationship.

Trust Your Instincts

Instincts are our internal guardians. When something in a relationship feels off, it often is. Trusting your gut might seem like an old cliché, but it's a powerful tool honed by millennia of human evolution. Your subconscious can pick up on inconsistencies and signals in someone's behavior before your conscious mind registers them. If you feel uneasy, if there's a little voice inside you raising a concern, listen to it. It's okay to take a step back and reassess. Remember, authentic connections can withstand scrutiny, and the pace of building trust should make both parties feel comfortable.

Role of Healthy Skepticism

Having a healthy level of skepticism is like having a sound immune system for your emotional health—it helps you ward off potential harm. In the context of new relationships, this means not taking everything at face value. Observe how the person behaves in various situations; do their actions align with their words? Are there inconsistencies that make you feel uneasy? Healthy skepticism encourages you to ask questions and seek understanding about whom the person truly is beyond the surface.

Early Boundary Setting

Setting boundaries early in any relationship is crucial. It's like laying down the rules of a game before you start playing: it ensures that everyone knows expectations and how to behave to keep things fair and enjoyable. Communicate your limits clearly and observe how they are respected (or not). Someone's reaction to your boundaries can tell you much about their respect for you.

If they push back, minimize your concerns, or ignore your boundaries altogether, these are clear indicators that they may not value your needs and autonomy as they should.

Navigating new relationships after experiencing abuse requires a blend of awareness, intuition, and assertiveness. By recognizing red flags, trusting your instincts, applying healthy skepticism, and setting boundaries early, you equip yourself with tools to protect your emotional well-being and open up to more nutritious, more fulfilling relationships. These strategies aren't about building walls but about installing clear, respectful gates that allow the right people into your life—those who will walk the garden with you, mindful not to trample the flowers.

8.5 Building Resilience: Strategies to Prevent Future Abuse

Resilience might conjure images of weather-beaten cliffs standing firm against the onslaught of raging seas. Still, in our context, it's about building an internal stronghold that guards against emotional storms. Think of resilience not just as bouncing back but as bouncing forward. It's about using the insight from previous experiences to fortify yourself against future encounters that might echo past abuses. Let's explore how enhancing self-awareness, educating yourself continuously, cultivating a supportive network, and mastering self-advocacy can serve as your armor and weapons in this ongoing battle for emotional safety and well-being.

Strengthening Self-Awareness

Self-awareness is like an internal compass; it helps you navigate your emotional landscape, understand where you are, and point toward where you need to go. Journaling and mindfulness help you chart your daily emotional experiences and highlight patterns that might make you vulnerable to future abuses. For instance, journaling can unveil tendencies to downplay your feelings or dismiss red flags, habits often shaped by past abusive dynamics. Through mindfulness, you can cultivate a heightened awareness of the present moment, allowing you to recognize and address these tendencies as they arise rather than letting them steer you unknowingly.

Mindfulness, in particular, teaches you to observe your thoughts and feelings without judgment—a crucial skill when untangling the complex emotions left by narcissistic abuse. It helps you sit with uncomfortable emotions, understand them, and eventually manage them without being overwhelmed. This ongoing practice fortifies your emotional resilience, making you less susceptible to old patterns of thinking and reacting that a narcissist might exploit.

Educational Empowerment

Knowledge is power, and in the context of narcissistic abuse, it's your shield. Educating yourself about narcissistic behaviors, understanding the psychological underpinnings of emotional abuse, and familiarizing yourself with healthy relationship dynamics can transform the way you perceive and react to potential violations. This education can come from books, articles, workshops, and even insightful documentaries. Each piece of information adds a layer of protection, helping you spot and sidestep behaviors previously unchecked.

Moreover, this continuous learning process empowers you to break the cycle of abuse. It shifts your role from a passive recipient of abuse to an active defender against it. Knowledge equips you with the tools to deconstruct manipulative tactics and rebuild your interactions on foundations of respect and mutual understanding. It ensures that the signs of potential abuse aren't unrecognized or unchallenged.

Building a Supportive Network

Survivors of narcissistic abuse often find themselves isolated, a condition carefully engineered by their abusers. Rebuilding, or in some cases, building a network of supportive, trustworthy people from scratch, is akin to constructing a lifeboat after surviving a shipwreck. This network should include individuals who can offer emotional support, provide healthy perspectives on relationships, and celebrate your victories, no matter how small.

Engaging in community activities, joining clubs or groups that align with your interests, or even volunteering are great options for meeting new people. These connections provide emotional buffers and a sense of belonging, reducing the feeling of loneliness that often accompanies recovery from abusive relationships. Remember, the goal is not to replace one dependency with another but to foster a community that supports your autonomy and growth.

Self-Advocacy Skills

Finally, the art of self-advocacy is like learning to speak a new language—the language of assertiveness. It involves expressing your needs and rights clearly and confidently, without apology or aggression. Self-advocacy is crucial in setting boundaries and maintaining them. It requires you to value your own needs as much as you might have been conditioned to prioritize the needs of the narcissist during the abusive relationship.

Practicing self-advocacy can start in small, everyday interactions—speaking up if you're overcharged at a store, for example, or expressing a preference in plans with friends. Each act of self-advocacy reinforces your belief in your worth and your right to be heard, setting the stage for stronger, more assertive responses in more significant relationships.

Building resilience against future abuse is a multifaceted endeavor. It encompasses deep self-awareness, continuous education, a supportive community, and robust self-advocacy skills. Together, these strategies weave a protective fabric around your emotional well-being, empowering you to navigate future relationships with confidence, discernment, and a profound sense of self-worth. As you continue to build and reinforce these strategies, remember that resilience isn't just about enduring; it's about thriving and transforming past pains into lessons and strengths that pave the way for a healthier, happier future.

8.6 New Beginnings: Embracing Hope and New Relationships

Think of this moment as standing at the threshold of a new house —your house—where every nook awaits your touch to turn it into a home. It's about stepping into new beginnings with a hopeful heart, a space where past lessons form the foundation of healthier, more fulfilling relationships. Embracing this positivity isn't about forgetting the past; instead, it's about applying the wisdom from those experiences to foster nurturing and genuine connections.

Imagine you're planting a garden. Each relationship is a seed, and your past experiences are the gardening skills you've honed—knowing which spots get the most sunlight, which plants need more water, and which soil is best. Like gardening, taking things slow in new relationships allows you to understand the environment better, ensuring that each new connection has the best chance to grow healthy and strong. Rushing this process can be tempting, especially when loneliness casts a long shadow, but remember, a tree that takes years to grow holds its ground far longer than one hastily planted.

Celebrating your personal growth becomes your daily ritual in this garden of new relationships. Each small act of self-care, every boundary set and respected, is a testament to your growth through your recovery journey. This celebration isn't just about moving past what happened but moving forward with a new sense of self-awareness and strength. These qualities transform not only how you view relationships but also how you engage in them. They allow you to bring your most authentic self to the table, creating connections that are not just about finding companionship but about mutual growth and support.

As you cultivate these new relationships, planning for the future is essential. Setting goals for what you want from your relationships and your personal life can act as your roadmap, helping you navigate through choices and challenges with clarity and purpose. Whether these goals are about achieving emotional intimacy, building trust, or simply learning to have fun again, they serve as guideposts, ensuring that every aligned step you take is toward your desires and values. This forward-thinking isn't just about making plans; it's about taking control of your narrative and crafting a future that resonates with who you are and aspire to be.

Through embracing positivity, taking things slow, celebrating your growth, and planning your future, you set the stage for relationships that bring joy, respect, and fulfillment. Remember, these new beginnings are not just about finding the right people to share your life with; they're about being the right person in your own life, one who is whole, healed, and ready to welcome new connections with open arms and a hopeful heart.

As this chapter closes, remember that each step has been a stepping stone to a stronger, more resilient you. The relationships you form now are reflections of your journey, mirrors that show not just where you've been but how far you've come. Embrace this new chapter with hope for the promise of something extraordinary in each new beginning. And as you turn the page, ready to write the next chapter, carry forward the lessons, the love, and the laughter that this journey has bestowed upon you.

Tailoring the Message

Your audience can vary widely—from victims just recognizing their situation to the general public curious about the topic to professionals seeking more in-depth understanding. Each group needs a different pitch. For victims, your tone should be gentle and validating, offering them the vocabulary to articulate their experiences. With the general public, aim for clarity and relatability; use everyday situations or popular media references to illustrate points. For professionals, bring in data, research, and case studies that provide a rigorous view of how widespread and damaging narcissism can be.

Imagine you're at a workshop. Your audience includes social workers, psychologists, and survivors. Your challenge is to weave your narrative to resonate with each subgroup. Start with a broad introduction, followed by personal stories for emotional impact (engaging survivors), then intersperse with statistics and studies (catering to professionals), and conclude with practical advice (helpful for social workers).

Educational Settings

The settings where you share your knowledge can vary from intimate workshops to seminars, online forums, and webinars. Each setting requires a different engagement strategy. In workshops, engage with interactive activities that allow participants to apply terms in role-play or scenario analysis. In seminars, use compelling visuals and narratives that highlight key points. Online, think about interactive polls or Q&A sessions to make the learning dynamic and responsive.

For example, in a webinar on identifying narcissistic behaviors, you could set up a live poll asking attendees to choose what action they would take in a hypothetical scenario involving a narcissistic coworker. This would make the session interactive and help attendees apply their learning in real time, testing their understanding and encouraging active participation.

Handling Misconceptions

Narcissism is often misunderstood. Some see it simply as self-love or confidence, but you know it's more perilous, especially when it crosses into abuse. Address these misconceptions head-on. When someone trivializes narcissism as just another personality quirk, counter with facts and personal stories that highlight its destructive impact. Use before-and-after scenarios to show how deeply narcissistic abuse can affect individuals, altering their perception of self and their interaction with the world.

For instance, if someone believes narcissistic behavior is just about being self-centered, explain the concept of 'narcissistic injury' and 'rage'—how a narcissist reacts to perceived slights with extreme responses affecting all around them. Illustrate this with a story, perhaps about a time when a simple disagreement led to disproportionate consequences, helping the listener see the seriousness of the condition.

Educating others about narcissism isn't just about spreading knowledge; it's about adjusting lenses, changing perspectives, and, sometimes, changing lives. As you share your understanding, remember that you're not just recounting facts; you're offering a map to those still navigating the labyrinth of narcissistic abuse. Your words have the power to validate, enlighten, and empower. Use them wisely, and watch as understanding blossoms where misconceptions once took root.

8.7 Advocacy and Change: Creating Awareness in Your Community

Roll up your sleeves because getting involved in community engagement is like organizing a neighborhood block party. You want everyone to come out, have a good time, and leave feeling a little more connected than they did before. But instead of grilling burgers and playing corn hole, you're raising awareness about narcissistic abuse—a topic that could potentially change lives.

Start by organizing local events. Consider setting up an information booth at the following street fair or hosting a talk at the local community center. These are not just opportunities to spread the word; they're also great ways to meet others passionate about mental health advocacy or who may need your information.

Participating in health fairs can also be a fruitful avenue. These events attract a diverse crowd eager to learn more about improving their well-being. By setting up a booth with engaging materials like brochures, interactive quizzes, and even a looping documentary snippet on narcissistic behaviors, you can educate people on recognizing these toxic patterns not just in their romantic relationships but in any social interaction. Collaborating with local mental health organizations can amplify your efforts. These organizations already have the infrastructure and the audience but lack detailed information on narcissism, which is where your insights become invaluable. Together, you can host workshops, support groups, or even training sessions for mental health professionals.

Regarding policy advocacy, think of yourself as a lobbyist for the heart. It's about taking your understanding of narcissistic abuse and turning it into actionable change that protects and empowers victims at the community or even state level. Learn how to connect with lawmakers—those folks who have the power to enact laws that recognize and protect against narcissistic abuse. Start small by attending town hall meetings or scheduling meetings with your local representatives to discuss potential changes in regulations or to introduce new policies that better support victims of narcissistic abuse.

Joining or forming advocacy groups can provide a collective, powerful voice. These groups often have leverage in policy discussions, representing a larger segment of the community. They also offer support, resources, and a network of like-minded individuals who can share strategies and successes from other areas. This can be invaluable when navigating the often complex landscape of public policy and lawmaking.

Building partnerships with local organizations, schools, and workplaces is crucial. These institutions are fundamental in shaping the community's understanding and response to narcissistic abuse —for instance, partnering with schools to integrate discussions on healthy relationships and emotional abuse into their curriculum. In workplaces, advocate for training sessions that help employees recognize and safely respond to narcissistic behaviors, which can often manifest in professional environments just as they do in personal ones.

Lastly, ensure your efforts have measurable impacts. Hosting an event is satisfying, but how do you know if it made a difference? Set clear, quantifiable goals for your advocacy efforts. You could aim to reach 100 people at a seminar or have 50 individuals sign up for more information. You may be pushing for a specific policy change by the end of the year. Whatever your goals, having these metrics helps maintain focus and provides concrete evidence of your impact—a crucial element when applying for grants or reporting back to stakeholders.

Advocating for change in your community can be a challenging yet gratifying endeavor. It's about more than just spreading information; it's about weaving a fabric of understanding and support that can fundamentally change how society recognizes and deals with narcissistic abuse. Every pamphlet handed out, every workshop conducted, and every policy change adds a thread to this fabric, strengthening the collective approach to dealing with narcissism and supporting those affected by it. So, get out there, connect, educate, and transform. Your voice and actions are not just dropped in the ocean—they're the currents that can steer our community toward safer, healthier interpersonal dynamics.

8.8 Using Your Experience to Help Others

Imagine sitting down with a friend over coffee, sharing stories of your experiences—the ups, the downs, and those pivotal moments that shaped your journey through narcissistic abuse. Now, think about the power these shared stories have—to mend your heart and to light a path for others who might still be searching for a way out of their darkness. Sharing your personal story isn't just about recounting events; it's about turning your past struggles into beacons of hope and tools for education.

When guiding others on how to share their personal stories, it's crucial to emphasize the balance between transparency and personal comfort. Start by choosing which parts of your story to share. Not every detail needs to be public. Pick moments that highlight significant insights about narcissistic abuse—those turning points where you learned something vital about yourself or the nature of your abuser. It's like selecting ingredients for a recipe; you want just enough to convey the flavor without overwhelming your audience.

However, while sharing, safeguarding your emotional health is paramount. Before you open up, gauge your emotional readiness. Are you comfortable discussing the details? Will it bring up trauma or empower you? Sometimes, sharing can rekindle painful emotions. It's okay to step back and heal more before sharing. If you're ready, consider starting in a small, supportive environment such as a therapy session, a support group, or a trusted friend.

These are spaces where vulnerability is accepted and embraced, providing a soft landing for the hard truths you share.

Transitioning into a mentorship role can be a natural next step. Mentoring allows you to use your past pain for a constructive purpose, guiding other survivors through the labyrinth of recovery that you once walked yourself. As a mentor, you can offer empathy, practical advice, and emotional support, tailoring your guidance to the specific needs and circumstances of those you're helping. Remember, mentoring is not just about giving; it's a reciprocal relationship. Each interaction offers insights and a chance to reflect on your growth, reinforcing your resilience and wisdom.

Start by observing if you're considering stepping into a mentor or support role within a group. Each group has its dynamics; understanding these can help you contribute effectively. When you're ready, share insights from your experiences that might resonate with the group. Your real-life examples can make abstract concepts of narcissistic abuse tangible, helping others see the patterns in their relationships. Also, be open to feedback. Support groups are collective healing spaces where everyone, including you, is there to grow.

Volunteering with organizations that advocate for abuse survivors can extend your impact even further. Extension of your impact could involve facilitating group meetings, organizing awareness campaigns, or providing one-on-one support. Each role offers unique opportunities to use your journey for a broader purpose. For instance, if you're artistically inclined, consider helping with marketing materials for a domestic abuse awareness campaign. If you're a natural organizer, perhaps coordinate events or workshops. Such involvement not only aids others but can also be incredibly healing for you, reaffirming your strength and agency.

Volunteering also opens pathways to connect with professionals and other volunteers who share your passion for advocacy. These connections can be enriching, offering new perspectives and ideas that can enhance your understanding and methods of support. Moreover, these roles often provide access to additional training and resources that can deepen your ability to help effectively, ensuring that informed and impactful actions match your good intentions.

As you step into these roles, whether sharing your story, mentoring, contributing to support groups, or volunteering, remember the dual purpose of your actions: to assist others and to continue your healing journey. Each story you share, each person you help, illuminates their path and reinforces the bridge you've built over your past challenges. In these acts of giving, you reaffirm your resilience and redefine your experiences, not as chains of the past but as wings for the future.

8.9 Resources and Tools for Ongoing Education

Let's chat about turning your newfound understanding of narcissism into a superpower, shall we? Think of it as arming yourself with a toolbox, where each other's design carves out a more straightforward path through the often misunderstood landscape of narcissistic abuse. To do this effectively, you need the best resources at your fingertips—books that open new windows of understanding, articles that challenge and refine your perspectives, and videos that bring abstract concepts into sharp, relatable focus. For starters, books like "Will I Ever Be Good Enough?" by Karyl McBride or "Disarming the Narcissist" by Wendy T. Behary offer deep dives into the mechanics of coping with and understanding narcissists. Articles, especially those found on platforms like Psychology Today, provide ongoing, up-to-date insights that can keep you informed about the latest research and strategies. Videos from channels like TEDx, where psychologists discuss the impacts of selfish behavior, can visually and emotionally connect you to the experiences and solutions shared by experts in the field.

Now, let's talk about beefing up your credentials. If you're feeling particularly inspired and wish to take this further, consider professional development opportunities such as conferences on mental health, psychology webinars, or even certifications in counseling that focus on narcissistic abuse recovery. These can transform your journey into a professional toolkit, enabling you to help others navigate this challenging terrain. Imagine attending a conference where you gain knowledge and connect with a community as passionate as you are about making a difference. Each seminar or workshop attended adds layers to your understanding, turning you into a beacon of hope and help for those still lost in the confusion of their experiences.

Online learning platforms are treasure troves of information and are wonderfully accessible. Websites like Coursera or Udemy offer psychology and mental health courses that can help you understand the broader nuances of human behavior and emotional manipulation. These platforms often feature courses designed by university professors and seasoned professionals, providing both depth and breadth of learning. Engaging in these courses allows you to learn at your own pace, revisit complex topics, and apply your knowledge in real-world scenarios, all from the comfort of your home.

Lastly, why not share your insights and experiences by creating content? Start a blog, launch a podcast, or even post about your journey and discoveries on social media. Each post can be a lifeline to someone silently struggling, and each podcast episode is a signpost guiding them toward understanding and recovery. Sharing content helps others and reinforces your learning and healing. It's a cycle of positive reinforcement, where teaching others teaches you, and healing others helps heal you. Plus, in creating content, you engage with a global community, learning from their feedback and perspectives, which, in turn, enriches your understanding.

Navigating through the resources and opportunities for education and sharing in the realm of narcissistic abuse is like piecing together a puzzle. Each book, article, video, course, and piece of content adds a piece to the bigger picture. As you learn, share, and grow, you empower yourself and light the way for others, turning your past experiences into a powerful catalyst for change and healing. Remember, every resource you engage with, every piece of knowledge you acquire, and every story you share adds to a collective understanding, forging paths of recovery and resilience for those affected by narcissistic abuse.

8.10 The Power of Storymaking: Sharing Your Journey

Think of storytelling as a form of art where each brushstroke adds color and depth to the canvas of your experiences. For both the storyteller and the audience, this art form has a magical way of weaving connections and fostering healing. When you share your journey, especially one as tumultuous as surviving narcissistic abuse, you're not just recounting events; you're offering a piece of yourself that can profoundly touch others, validating their experiences and encouraging them to embrace their healing paths. It's like opening a window in a stuffy room—the fresh air doesn't just benefit you; it revitalizes everyone in the space.

Storytelling is therapeutic because it helps you, the storyteller, organize your thoughts, process your emotions, and make sense of the chaos that once seemed to dominate your life. It's a method of reclaiming your narrative and moving from a place of pain to power. For the audience, whether they are survivors themselves or simply empathetic listeners, your story can be a beacon of hope or a bridge to understanding. It illuminates the invisible wounds of emotional abuse, making them feel less alone in their struggles. Moreover, it can be empowering, showing them that recovery isn't just possible but within their grasp.

Crafting Your Story

When you decide to share your story, think of it as crafting a journey for your audience. Begin where you feel your journey began. Was it the first moment you recognized something was wrong or when you finally decided to seek help? From there, build towards pivotal moments—these are your plot points. Maybe it was a particularly painful instance of gaslighting or perhaps a moment of clarity where you saw the truth. These moments should build towards a climax, the turning point. For many, this might be the moment of leaving or an essential realization that changed everything.

As you lay out these events, develop your characters, which will likely include yourself and the narcissist in your story. Show your growth, your struggles, and your victories. Paint the narcissist realistically—resist the temptation to demonize, as the truth of their actions will speak loudly enough. Setting scenes is equally important. Bring your audience into the environments where your story unfolded. Describe the cold, unwelcoming kitchen where arguments happened or the cozy coffee shop where you planned your escape. These details aren't just filler; they ground your story in reality, making it relatable and immersive.

Platforms for Sharing

Now, where to share your story? The platforms are as varied as the stories themselves. If you're comfortable with public speaking, consider sharing at events focused on mental health, community gatherings, or workshops. These venues allow for immediate interaction and can be profoundly impactful for both you and your audience. If you prefer writing, a memoir or a series of blog posts can be therapeutic. They allow you to structure your thoughts and reach a broader audience, often beyond your immediate community.

For those who enjoy social media's connectivity, creating video content or podcasts can be powerful. These mediums combine personal storytelling with wide reach, engaging people through visuals and voices, making the experience more personal. Remember, each platform has nuances, so tailor your story to fit the medium. For instance, a blog post can be reflective and detailed, while a podcast might be more conversational.

Protecting Privacy

In all this, protecting your privacy is paramount. Not all details need to be shared, and it's okay to change names or details to safeguard your identity and the identities of others. Decide in advance which aspects of your story are off-limits, and stick to these boundaries. It's also wise to consider the potential impact of your story on your personal and professional life, especially if shared publicly. Sometimes, sharing under a pseudonym or focusing more on the lessons learned rather than specific details can be effective ways to maintain privacy while offering support and insight to others.

In essence, sharing your journey through storytelling is not just about unburdening yourself or educating others; it's a profound act of connection and healing. It's a way to take the scattered pieces of your past, assemble them into a coherent narrative, and offer them up to the world not as a tale of victimhood but as a story of survival and strength. As you share, remember that each word, pause, and breath is a step toward personal relief, communal understanding, and healing. Your story is not just your own; it is a shared human experience, resonating with universal themes of pain, resilience, and the enduring hope for a brighter tomorrow.

8.11 Future Trends in Understanding and Teaching Narcissistic Abuse

As we peer into the horizon of psychological research and treatment, it feels a bit like standing on the cusp of a technological revolution, but for mental health. The landscape of understanding narcissism and treating its repercussions is evolving rapidly, driven by new research, technological advancements, and a growing global perspective on mental health.

Emerging Research

First, let's dive into the latest buzz from the research world. Scientists and psychologists are tirelessly piecing together the complex puzzle that is narcissism. Recent studies are focusing on the neurobiological underpinnings of narcissistic behaviors, which could revolutionize how we approach treatment. Imagine treatments targeted not just the symptoms but the neural activities that underlie these behaviors. This treatment could lead to more effective interventions tailored to the individual rather than the one-size-fits-all approach we often see today.

Moreover, researchers are exploring the impact of early childhood experiences in shaping narcissistic traits. This line of inquiry holds the promise of early intervention strategies that could prevent the full-blown development of narcissistic personality disorder. It's akin to planting a healthier garden by understanding the best conditions and care from the seedling stage—nurturing resilience and empathy before the weeds of narcissism take root.

Technological Advancements

Next, let's talk tech. The digital age is transforming how we manage and recover from narcissistic abuse. Virtual reality (VR) therapies, for instance, are on the cutting edge, offering safe spaces for survivors to confront their experiences and practice responses to narcissistic behaviors in a controlled, virtual environment. Imagine donning a VR headset and role-playing scenarios where you assert boundaries or practice self-affirmation, all guided by a therapist, without ever facing real-world repercussions.

Apps and online therapies are making waves, too, democratizing access to support and resources. These platforms provide anonymity and accessibility, which is crucial for those who might feel isolated or stigmatized by their experiences. They offer everything from daily affirmations and mindfulness exercises to chats with therapists and support groups, all at your fingertips. It's like having a therapist in your pocket, ready to help whenever and wherever you need it.

Global Perspectives

The global dialogue on narcissism is expanding as well. Cultural differences in recognizing and treating narcissistic abuse are being more widely acknowledged and addressed. What works in one cultural context may not work in another, and the global mental health community is working towards more culturally sensitive approaches. Collaborations across countries and cultures enrich the resources available, whether through shared research, international conferences, or cross-cultural therapy practices. This exchange enhances our understanding and ensures a more holistic approach to tackling narcissistic abuse.

Predictions and Preparations

So, what's on the horizon? We can expect a continued push towards personalized mental health care, where genetic, neural, and psychological data all play a role in crafting individual treatment plans. Community-based interventions might also see a rise, with increased emphasis on preventing narcissistic abuse through community education and support systems.

Staying informed about these trends is crucial for those navigating life post-narcissism or for professionals in the field. It prepares you to make the most of new tools and understandings as they become available. It also empowers you to participate in shaping the future dialogue on narcissistic abuse, ensuring that it remains inclusive, informed, and innovative.

As we wrap up this exploration of future trends, it's clear that the journey toward understanding and treating narcissistic abuse is one of collaboration, innovation, and hope. The landscape is changing, and with each new development, we move closer to a world where recovery is possible and supported by the best tools science and technology offer. Let's carry this spirit of innovation and empathy into the next chapter, where we'll explore personal stories of resilience and recovery, weaving together the insights and strategies we've discussed into a tapestry of empowerment and healing.

Thank You for Reading!

I hope you found this book on understanding and dealing with narcissism helpful. Your feedback is incredibly valuable to me and helps other readers discover this book.

If you enjoyed this book or found it useful, **please consider leaving a review on Amazon.** It only takes a few minutes, and your review will help me improve my work and reach more readers who may benefit from this information.

Scan Me

Conclusion

As we draw the curtains on this journey—our shared exploration into the shadowed valleys and sunlit paths of understanding and healing from narcissistic abuse—I want to take a moment to reflect on the ground we've covered together. From the early chapters, where we decoded the complexities of narcissism, to the empowering strategies for setting boundaries and fostering self-love, we've navigated some rugged terrain. You've learned to survive and thrive beyond the reach of toxic influences.

The essence of our journey underscores a powerful truth: self-love and firm boundaries are not just shields but also the foundation upon which we rebuild ourselves. By embracing these principles, you arm yourself against future emotional turmoil, ensuring that your path forward is one you walk with confidence and clarity.

As we've seen, knowledge is more than power—it's protection. Understanding the red flags of narcissism, the subtle signs of manipulation, and the psychological underpinnings of toxic behavior equips you to recognize and sidestep potential hazards in your relational landscape. Hold on to this knowledge; let it guide you as you progress.

But don't stop here. I encourage you to keep the flames of education and advocacy burning. Share your insights, speak out in your communities, and help illuminate the shadows of narcissistic abuse for others. Each conversation and shared story adds to a collective beacon of awareness and change.

Remember, the road to recovery is steeped in challenges but also ripe with opportunities for profound personal growth and transformation. You are different from the person who started this book. You are more robust, wiser, and equipped with the tools to survive and soar above the legacy of past abuses.

Building and leaning on a support network can make all the difference. Whether it's friends who offer a listening ear, family who provide a comforting presence, or professionals who guide you through the complexities of healing, remember you're never alone. These connections are vital, giving support, reflections on your progress, and reminders of your resilience.

And to you, brave reader, I commend your strength and courage. Stepping into the light of truth, especially when it reveals the painful realities of narcissism, is no small feat. Remember this moment and how far you've come if you ever doubt your journey. For those moments that feel overwhelmingly complex, never hesitate to seek professional help. Therapy isn't just a remedy; it's a tool for transformation—an investment in your future self.

As we part ways in this book, know you're not stepping out alone. You are part of a vibrant, ever-expanding community of survivors and advocates, each of us walking our paths but guided by shared lights of hope and healing. Carry forward the message of this book, not just as a survivor of narcissistic abuse but as a beacon of resilience and a champion of your own story.

Together, we are stronger. Together, we heal, we grow, and we transcend. Thank you for sharing this journey with me. May your path forward be bright, and always find light in the shadows.

References

100 Positive Affirmations For Abuse Survivors (Heal Fast!) https://thegoodpositive.com/positive-affirmations-for-abuse-survivors/

21 Signs of Emotional Abuse in Relationships https://psychcentral.com/lib/emotionalabuse-signs

5 Powerful Self-Care Tips for Abuse and Trauma Survivors https://www.thehotline.org/resources/5-powerful-self-care-tips-for-abuse-and-trauma-survivors/

5 Steps to Heal From Emotional Abuse https://www.psychologytoday.com/us/blog/hopefor-relationships/202311/5-steps-to-heal-from-emotional-abuse

6 Steps to Communicating with Toxic People Effectively https://institute.uschamber.com/6-steps-to-communicating-with-toxic-people-effectively/

6 Traits of Covert Narcissism https://health.clevelandclinic.org/covert-narcissism

Advocacy in mental health - PMC https://www.ncbi.nlm.nih.gov/pmc/articles/PMC8793719/

Effective Communication: Improving Your Interpersonal Skills https://www.helpguide.org/articles/relationships-communication/effective-communication.htm

Emotional Abuse Laws https://www.legalmatch.com/law-library/article/emotional-abuse-laws.html

Financial Planning Before, During and After a Divorce https://smartasset.com/financial-advisor/divorce-financial-planning

Gaslighting: What it is, long-term effects, and what to do https://www.medicalnewstoday.com/articles/long-term-effects-of-gaslighting

Grey rock method: What it is and how to use it effectively https://www.medicalnewstoday.com/articles/grey-rock

Healing From Narcissistic Abuse https://www.verywellmind.com/stages-of-healingafter-narcissistic-abuse-5207997

How Intentional Solitude Can Work To Heal Your ... https://medium.com/the-partneredpen/how-intentional-solitude-can-work-to-heal-your-emotional-wounds-cf02dbe5acb6

How to Break Free From a Trauma Bond https://www.psychologytoday.com/us/blog/the-angry-therapist/202310/how-to-break-free-from-a-trauma-bond

How to Get Out of an Abusive Relationship https://www.helpguide.org/articles/abuse/getting-out-of-an-abusive-relationship.htm

References

How to Heal From Emotional Abuse: The Ultimate Guide To ... https://eddinscounseling.com/how-to-heal-from-emotional-abuse/

How to Set Boundaries With a Narcissist | Charlie Health https://www.charliehealth.com/post/how-to-set-boundaries-with-a-narcissist

How to Use Mindfulness to Ease and Heal Trauma https://www.healthline.com/health/how-trauma-informed-mindfulness-helps-me-heal-from-the-past-and-cope-with-the-present

Long-Term Effects of Narcissistic Abuse - Charlie Health https://www.charliehealth.com/post/the-long-term-effects-of-narcissistic-abuse

Melanie Tonia Evans - Narcissistic Abuse Recovery https://melanietoniaevans.com/

Narcissistic Abuse: Examples, Signs, and Effects https://www.talkspace.com/mentalhealth/conditions/articles/narcissistic-abuse/

Narcissistic Personality Disorder in Clinical ... https://www.ncbi.nlm.nih.gov/pmc/articles/PMC5819598/

Narcissistic Rage: Identifying & Protecting Yourself https://www.talkspace.com/mentalhealth/conditions/articles/narcissistic-rage/

National Domestic Violence Hotline: Domestic Violence Support https://www.thehotline.org/

New Insights Into Narcissistic Personality Disorder https://www.psychiatrictimes.com/view/new-insights-narcissistic-personality-disorder#:

Support groups: Make connections, get help https://www.mayoclinic.org/healthy-life-style/stress-management/in-depth/support-groups/art-20044655

Victims of domestic violence - New York State Attorney General https://ag.ny.gov/publications/victims-domestic-violence#:

What Is The Best Therapy for Narcissistic Abuse? https://www.charliehealth.com/post/what-is-the-best-therapy-for-narcissistic-abuse

When Letting Go Is Tough: How to Emotionally Detach from ... https://psychcentral.com/lib/the-what-why-when-and-how-of-detaching-from-loved-ones

Made in the USA
Las Vegas, NV
29 April 2025

21498506R00079